- Do you feel moody and uncomfortable during the time before your period?
- Do you suffer from skin disorders such as eczema or psoriasis?
- Are you crippled by asthma or arthritis?
- Are you looking for a way to lower your cholesterol and blood pressure?
- Are you worried about the dangers or side effects of taking prescription medications?
- Would you like help losing weight?

IF YOU ANSWERED "YES" TO ANY OF THESE QUESTIONS, LEARN THE SECRETS OF ONE OF THE MOST POPULAR HERBAL SUPPLEMENTS ON THE MARKET. LEARN THE SECRETS OF EVENING PRIMROSE OIL

SECRETS
of Evening
Primrose Oil

MONICA REINAGEL

A LYNN SONBERG BOOK

St. Martin's Paperbacks

SECRETS OF EVENING PRIMROSE OIL

Copyright © 2000 by Lynn Sonberg Book Associates.

ISBN: 0-312-97298-9

Printed in the United States of America

St. Martin's Paperbacks edition / February 2000

10 9 8 7 6 5 4 3 2

IMPORTANT NOTE:

This book is for informational purposes only. It is not intended to take the place of medical advice from a trained medical professional. Readers are advised to consult a physician or other qualified health professional regarding treatment of all of their health problems or before acting on any of the information or advice in this book.

This book is intended to provide selected information about evening primrose oil. Research about evening primrose oil is ongoing and subject to conflicting interpretations. As a result, there is no guarantee that what we know about this subject will not change with time.

Contents

Introduction

OVER a century ago, the seed of a common wild-flower, the evening primrose, was found to contain an unusual oil with remarkable health-restoring abilities. In this book you will learn the many secrets of evening primrose oil (EPO), one of the most versatile and therapeutic nutritional supplements ever discovered. Benefits of this unlikely nutritional superstar range from relief from premenstrual syndrome, to lowering high cholesterol and high blood pressure, to alleviating suffering from rheumatoid arthritis and multiple sclerosis. It also has been used successfully to treat allergies, asthma, skin disorders, schizophrenia, alcoholism, and obesity.

It might seem unlikely that this long list of seemingly unrelated conditions could all be improved by a single nutritional supplement. In fact, some people have dismissed the powers attributed to evening primrose oil as the claims of snake oil salesmen. In truth, the explanation is quite simple and firmly grounded in biochemical science. As you will learn in this book, all of these health problems share a common denominator. Research has revealed that many of today's most frequent and vexing health conditions are related to essential fatty acid deficiency.

With one in three Americans classified as obese, it may seem ridiculous to suggest that a lack of fat is one of the culprits in our nation's deteriorating health. After all, we've spent the last several decades trying to *avoid* fat. In the 1970s, fat was singled out as the number-one culprit in the nation's heart disease epidemic. Millions banished butter from the family dining table and replaced it with "heart-healthy" margarine. Then, in the 1980s, "fat-free" became the mantra of the booming weight-loss industry, and reduced-fat and fat-free foods became the fastest-growing sector of the packaged foods market.

Ironically, as we later discovered, the artificially hydrogenated fats in margarine turned out to be a far greater threat to our hearts than the butter we were so conscientiously trying to avoid. And a decade-long binge on potatoes, pasta, and reduced-fat ice cream, cookies, and sweets left Americans disillusioned and heavier than ever. Too little fat and too many highly processed carbohydrates turned out to be a disastrous combination—and not just for dieters.

Now we are beginning to understand that while too much fat can be unhealthy, certain fats are absolutely critical for good health—and dangerously absent from our modern, highly processed food supplies. Adding the *right* fats to your diet is actually one of the best nutritional things you can do for your heart. And you might be surprised to learn that certain fats can *promote* weight loss without dieting. Evening primrose oil offers these and many other important nutritional and therapeutic benefits.

FORTY YEARS OF RESEARCH

The scientific literature contains thousands of pages of research on evening primrose oil. Hundreds of clinical studies have evaluated it in the treatment of conditions including eczema, premenstrual syndrome (PMS), fibrocystic (benign) breast disease, rheumatoid arthritis, heart disease, schizophrenia, alcoholism, cancer, and more. Unfortunately, the mainstream medical community, with its distinct pharmaceutical bias, often is slow to recognize and accept the medicinal properties of natural substances.

Despite the accumulated evidence in support of evening primrose oil, some researchers have been disdainful and dismissive of its "alleged benefits," citing studies that found "absolutely no evidence of any benefit." Upon further examination, many of these studies were conducted using low dosages that could not have been expected to produce positive results. Others studies lasted for too short a time for benefits to be ascertained, and still others inadvertently mixed the active ingredient with preservatives or other agents that blocked its absorption. While each of these studies provided valuable information, none of them really succeeded in doing what the authors had apparently set out to do, namely, to debunk the claims surrounding evening primrose oil.

A large part of the research conducted on evening primrose oil over the last thirty years was sponsored by the Efamol Research Institute in Nova Scotia, Canada, an affiliate of Efamol, Ltd., one of the world's largest producers of pharmaceutical-grade evening primrose oil. The company's involvement in both research and commerce has caused some to question the validity of the results—even data accepted for publication by peer-reviewed scientific journals. Unfortunately, this illustrates a classic Catch-22 faced by those in the natural products industry. On one hand, companies that promote natural products often are accused of making unsubstantiated claims on behalf of their products. On the other, when a company invests in scientific research to document the effectiveness of its product, the objectivity of the results is called into question. (Apparently what is acceptable operating procedure for pharmaceutical companies is biased self-interest if your product is a natural one.)

Efamol, Ltd., should be given credit for having plowed an enormous share of its revenue into scientific research that has considerably advanced the general knowledge and understanding of essential fats and the role they play in health. Much of the research has been corroborated by objective researchers unaffiliated with the company. Efamol also has published the results of trials that failed to demonstrate positive benefits.

Taken as a whole, the scientific research on evening primrose oil clearly demonstrates that this natural product offers significant health benefits. But that's only one part of the evidence. In our reverence for double-blind, placebo-controlled trials, we often overlook or undervalue another form of evidence, namely the cumulative clinical experience of physicians and just plain people who have been using evening primrose oil for decades with great success. Much of the information on clinical applications of evening primrose oil comes from Britain, where it has been widely prescribed for several decades as a treatment for premenstrual syndrome, fibrocystic (benign) breast disease, eczema, and multiple sclerosis.

In the relatively short time since it has become more widely available in the United States, evening primrose oil has risen to become one of the ten most popular nutritional supplements in the country, largely without benefit of large-scale marketing or advertising campaigns. Perhaps it is time to give the average consumer a little more credit. After all, hype or rumor might create a short-term interest in a new product, but if a product isn't effective, interest will soon fade. It's clear that people use evening primrose oil for the simple reason that it works. Women find that it relieves menstrual cramps, PMS, and breast pain. Arthritis sufferers find that they can decrease their reliance on pain medications. Doctors report reduced blood pressure and cholesterol levels in their patients who take evening primrose oil. People with asthma and eczema often can reduce their use of steroids and other medications. Weight may drop off effortlessly, and chronic acne can be transformed into a smooth and beautiful complexion.

This book reviews the scientific research, explains exactly how evening primrose oil works in the body, and shows you how it can be used in complete nutritional wellness programs for many common diseases and disorders. You'll also learn how to select the best sources of evening primrose oil and how to use it for maximum benefit.

Important note: The material in this book is provided for purpose of information only. It is not intended to take the place of advice from your doctor or qualified health practitioner. Please include your doctor in your decision to add evening primrose oil or any nutritional supplement to your daily regimen.

1

Down the Primrose Path

IT'S not hard to get excited about evening primrose oil . . . in fact, it has quite the Cinderella story. Until early in this century, the remarkable little evening primrose was regarded as little more than a common weed, growing uncultivated throughout North America and the United Kingdom. Almost by chance, it was discovered that the seed of this unassuming wildflower contains an oil quite unlike anything else in the animal or vegetable kingdom. Since its discovery, the unique healing properties of evening primrose oil have been the subject of decades of intense research by biochemists, medical researchers, physicians, and nutritionists the world over. Widely used in the British Isles for several decades, evening primrose oil now has become one of the most popular nutritional supplements in the United States and Canada, for reasons that will become evident throughout this book.

The evening primrose is not even a true primrose but is actually a member of the willow herb family, indigenous to the North American continent. Standing about three feet tall, the plant produces large, delicate yellow flowers that bloom for only a single night before withering. Not choosy about its habitat, the evening primrose will flourish even in the poorest, sandy soil. You will find this hardy wildflower growing along streams, roadsides, and beaches as well as in the desert plains, several thousand feet above sea level. In his book *What Herbs Are All About*, herbalist Jack Challem recounts his first encounter with the evening primrose: "They looked at first like tissue paper strewn across the desert. I had to stop because it looked like someone had littered the desert."

Native Americans valued the evening primrose as a medicinal herb of many talents. It was used to treat rashes and other inflammations of the skin, to heal wounds, to soothe whooping cough and tuberculosis, and as a sedative, diuretic, painkiller, and antispasmodic. English colonists of the New World learned of the medicinal properties of the evening primrose from Native Americans and promptly exported it to England, where it became known as King's Cure-all. Throughout the seventeenth and eighteenth centuries, the primrose was studied and prized as a versatile healer by European and North American herbalists.

Following its official introduction to Europe, the evening primrose proved to be a sturdy and willing traveler. Common to the sandy coastlines of North

America, seeds of the wild plants ended up mixed in with sand and soil used as ballast to weigh down cargo ships bearing cotton from the New World. This ballast was dumped on arrival at European ports, sowing the evening primrose wherever the ships landed. As sea trade between Europe and the United States flourished, the evening primrose proliferated throughout the European continent. To this day, it is seen growing wild along the coasts and port towns of Europe. Like many folk remedies, the evening primrose was known by numerous other names, including sand lily, tree primrose, rockrose, night willow, and German ranpion.

REDISCOVERING A FORGOTTEN TREASURE

By the beginning of the twentieth century, however, the evening primrose had largely fallen into disuse as a medicinal plant, although it continued to flourish in the wild. In 1917 a German scientist studying the properties of different vegetable oils first extracted and analyzed the oil from the seeds of the evening primrose and found that it contained a type of fatty acid that had never been seen before. The newly discovered molecule, of which the evening primrose seed was the only known source, was named gamma-linolenic acid (GLA), but it would be another half century before the significance of this discovery became apparent.

In the 1960s British researchers set out to determine what effects, if any, GLA might have on the body. By this time it was known that certain vegetable fats were necessary for the body to function properly. If animals were completely deprived of these essential fatty acids, or EFAs, certain symptoms of deficiency would develop, including hair loss and skin disorders. These symptoms could be reversed in relatively short order with the administration of vegetable oils that contained an essential fatty acid called linoleic acid.

Early research into the properties of GLA found that it could reverse the symptoms of essential fatty acid deficiency even more quickly than linoleic acid. This was somewhat surprising because GLA is not widely found in the food supply and was not considered to be an essential nutrient. But for some reason, the body seemed to use GLA more efficiently than linoleic acid. Biochemists later determined that the GLA found in evening primrose oil was up to ten times more biologically active.

Most of this early research into the properties of evening primrose oil was conducted under the auspices of a small British company by a staff biochemist named John Williams. This promising research was abruptly suspended when Williams's company was acquired by a large pharmaceutical company that did not intend to pursue further development of natural products. At this point, the odyssey of the evening primrose from sandlot weed to best-selling supplement might have faltered, if not for Williams's vision and commitment. Believing strongly in the potential of evening primrose oil as a natural pharmaceutical, Williams left the larger firm to start his own company. Bio Oil Research became the first firm to market evening primrose as a nutritional supplement, under the trade name Naudicell. Proceeds from the sale of the supplement funded further research into the biological activity of evening primrose oil.

EVENING PRIMROSE OIL COMES INTO ITS OWN

In the early 1970s a few researchers began studying the effects of essential fatty acids on various disease conditions. They reported that large amounts of sunflower seed oil, which is rich in linoleic acid, had the ability to halt or slow the progression of multiple sclerosis, a degenerative neurological disease. With few medical options for treating this devastating disease, people suffering from multiple sclerosis began to use sunflower oil. Those involved in the research on GLA and its superior bioactivity speculated that, if sunflower seed offered some benefit, evening primrose oil would be even more effective. Thus multiple sclerosis became the first condition for which evening primrose oil was widely used therapeutically.

While the reputation and popularity of evening primrose oil as a natural healer grew, researchers found that it had beneficial effects on blood cholesterol and blood pressure, suggesting its use in the treatment or prevention of heart disease. By the late 1970s, evening primrose oil had attracted the attention of other research biologists and biochemists, and the pace of research accelerated. A second company, Efamol Ltd., was formed and began to market evening primrose oil under the trade name Efamol. Now that the demand for evening primrose oil is well-established, many other manufacturers have entered the marketplace with EPO products of varying quality.

Under the direction of biochemist Dr. David Horrobin, the Efamol company sponsored extensive, ongoing research, coordinating over a hundred clinical trials of evening primrose oil in the treatment of dozens of serious health conditions. It was found that evening primrose oil could ease inflammation, modulate disturbed mood states, and resolve skin problems. Along the way, it also was discovered more or less inadvertently that evening primrose oil appeared to promote weight loss and prevent hangovers! The investigation gradually expanded to include an ever-widening array of uses for evening primrose oil, including employment as an antiviral agent and potential cancer-fighting agent.

The natural GLA content of the oil gets the credit for all of the curative and therapeutic powers of evening primrose oil. As researchers have discovered, GLA promotes the production of prostaglandins, hormonelike chemicals that regulate a host of critical cellular functions. Without enough GLA, prostaglandin production declines, and our health suffers. But why is such an important nutrient almost absent from our natural diet? The body is designed to make its own GLA out of linoleic acid, which, unlike GLA, is quite plentiful in our food supply. Under ideal circumstances, our diet should supply more than enough linoleic acid for the body to manufacture all the GLA it needs. However, as you'll see in the next chapter, many things can get in the way of this important process. Chronic stress, disease, poor diet, age, and the lack of certain nutrients in our diet can hinder our ability to process linoleic acid into GLA. A growing number of researchers and doctors now believe that many of the health conditions that plague us today can be traced to a deficiency of GLA in our bodies. Evening primrose oil steps into the gap, as a rich source of biologically active, preformed GLA.

The Many Benefits of Evening Primrose Oil

Acne   Helps prevent outbreaks

Alcoholism   Decreases withdrawal symptoms, improves liver function

Asthma and Allergy   Reduces allergic sensitivity

Dry Eyes   Helps with Sjögren's syndrome; also makes contact lenses more comfortable

Eczema   Reduces itching, redness, and inflammation. Reduces need for steroid medications

Fibrocystic (benign) Breast Disease   Reduces breast pain and tenderness, and cyst formation

High Blood Pressure   Lowers blood pressure

High Cholesterol   Lowers cholesterol levels and improves cholesterol ratios

Multiple Sclerosis Reduces severity and frequency of relapses

Obesity Promotes weight loss without dieting for those more than 10 percent overweight

PMS Reduces PMS symptoms, including mood swings, weight gain, and water retention

Rheumatoid Arthritis Reduces pain and inflammation. Reduces need for pain medication

Schizophrenia Improves depression, withdrawal, mental disturbance

---

It's interesting to note that although GLA is not commonly found in our diet, human breast milk is one of the richest known sources of this fatty acid. Babies have a particularly high requirement for fatty acids, which support the rapid growth and development of skin, bones, and organs and help to develop the newborn's immune system. It is well known that babies who are not breast-fed suffer from higher incidence of allergy, eczema, ear infections, and other maladies. In fact, many of the health problems seen in formula-fed babies correspond to conditions that evening primrose oil has been found to improve. Although infant formulas are designed to resemble human milk as closely as possible, formula manufacturers have overlooked the importance of these critical fatty acids. Recently Japanese manufacturers have begun fortifying baby formula with GLA and other important fatty acids, a trend that, it is hoped, will be copied in other parts of the world. In the meantime, all of us can reap the benefits of GLA in the form of evening primrose oil. Some have even called evening primrose oil "mother's milk for grown-ups."

Before we begin to examine the use of evening primrose in specific health conditions, the next chapter explains how GLA and other fatty acids work in the body and how the various types of fats in our diet affect our health.

2

The Secret of Evening Primrose Oil

AFTER decades of fat phobia, nutritionists are now beginning to recognize that certain fats are as essential to good health as vitamins and minerals. As the research has shown, evening primrose oil is a prime example of the critical role that healthful fats play in restoring health and wellness. We know that the gamma-linolenic acid (GLA) content in evening primrose oil is responsible for the many health benefits it offers. This chapter explains in more detail exactly how GLA works in the body to produce these many benefits. But first, let's untangle the somewhat confusing web of information about fats and how they can help or harm you.

THE GREAT FAT DEBATE

Despite the fact that we all need fats to be well, fat has somehow become public enemy number one, blamed for the epidemic rates of heart disease, obesity, and cancer that plague our modern society. For the last three decades, major public and private health agencies, including the U.S. Department of Agriculture, the American Heart Association, the National Cancer Institute as well as the popular media and the booming weight-loss industry have been encouraging Americans to reduce their fat intake. Some well-known weight-loss and heart-health experts have taken fat phobia to extremes, promoting a fat intake of as little as 10 percent of your daily calories.

The message has been rather one-sided: Fat is bad for you. And although fat consumption has decreased slightly in the past decade, we still consume on average about 35 percent of our daily calories as fat—only now we feel guilty about it. As you'll see later in this book, the fact is that low-fat diets are *not* an effective way to lose weight, nor are they the best way of preventing heart disease. Not only are the health benefits of extremely low-fat diets debatable, but such diets overlook a very important point: Fat is absolutely critical to proper body function.

MAKING FRIENDS WITH FAT

Fats are absolutely necessary for life. In addition to providing a concentrated source of calories—or energy—for every kind of physical activity, fat surrounds your vital internal organs, providing cushioning and insulation for these delicate parts. Body fat also helps us to conserve body heat and regulate body temperature. We need fat to deliver the fat-soluble vitamins (vitamins A, D, E, and K) to the cells of the body and to lubricate our intestines, facilitating elimination.

Every cell in the body is surrounded by a fatty membrane that helps the cell absorb the nutrients it needs while keeping out unwanted material. This fat, or *lipid*, membrane keeps cells flexible and slippery, which is especially important for blood (and other cells) that need to move easily throughout the body. Fats are very important to the skin cells (including the hair and nails), providing both moisture and waterproofing. The brain itself is composed of over 60 percent fat, which is critical to the production of neurotransmitters and for the transmission of nerve impulses that control everything from our heartbeat to our enjoyment of a beautiful sunset. A layer of fat called the myelin sheath insulates the brain and spinal cord, ensuring that the bioelectric signals that course through our nervous system arrive at their destinations intact and unscrambled. Finally, fats are a source of vitaminlike nutrients known as *essential fatty acids* (EFAs), which our bodies need in order to carry out basic biological functions.

The antifat campaign was well meaning, if misguided. After all, some research suggests that people who eat more fat tend to have higher risks of many diseases, notably our nation's number one and two killers, heart disease and cancer. But this may have been a gross oversimplification of the story. We now know that *what kind* of fat you eat is at least as important as *how much*. The problem is not just that we eat too much fat but, more specifically, that we eat too much of the wrong kinds of fat and not nearly enough of the right kinds. As hard as it may be to believe, many of today's most common health problems, such as those discussed later in this book, are the result of a *deficiency* of healthful fats, such as evening primrose oil.

Thankfully, we're finally beginning to emerge from the Dark Ages of fat phobia to a more sophisticated understanding of our complex nutritional needs. We're beginning to understand, for example, that all carbohydrates are not equally healthful. While complex carbohydrates such as whole grains and vegetables are high in vitamins, nutrients, and fiber, simple carbohydrates such as white bread, sweetened cereals, and packaged snacks have very little to offer nutritionally and can have a negative impact on health.

The same is true with dietary fats. Some fats, such as olive oil, fish oil, and evening primrose oil, provide nutrients that are absolutely essential for good health. Others, such as the saturated fats found in meat and dairy products, do not offer the same benefits. Even worse, certain fats, such as the hydrogenated oils found in margarine, mayonnaise, bottled salad dressing, and many snack foods, are downright damaging to our health.

Fat phobia has given way to a more balanced

view of fats and their relationship to health. The bottom line is this: We can dramatically reduce our risk of disease and improve our overall health by decreasing our intake of unhealthful fats and increasing our consumption of healthful fats. It's also a good idea to keep total fat calories to around 30 to 35 percent of our daily intake, in order to make sure we're also getting enough protein and other vital nutrients, such as the fiber, vitamins, and minerals found in naturally low-fat foods such as fruit, vegetables, and whole grains. The next section explains the different types of fat and how they function in the body.

THE FAMILY OF FATS

Dietary fats are usually sorted into three categories: saturated, monounsaturated, and polyunsaturated. Recently a fourth man-made category called trans fats has been added to the list. This categorization is determined by what kind of fatty acids are in the fats. All fats consist of building blocks called fatty acids, which are simply molecules of carbon, hydrogen, and oxygen arranged in a variety of configurations. The various fatty acids are considered to be saturated or unsaturated depending on the way the carbon, hydrogen, and oxygen atoms are connected to one another. Each of the different fatty acids functions differently in the body.

The Family of Fats

Saturated
Butter, Cream, Milk fat, Animal fat, Coconut oil, Palm oil, Palm kernel oil

Monounsaturated
Olive oil, Canola oil, Avocado oil

Polyunsaturated
Omega-3 (Linolenic Acid)
Fish oil, Flaxseed oil, Canola oil, Walnut oil, Soybean oil

Omega-6 (Alpha-linolenic Acid)
Corn oil, Safflower oil, Sunflower oil, Cottonseed oil, Soybean oil, Peanut oil, Sesame oil, Grapeseed oil, Borage oil, Evening primrose oil

Trans fats
Hydrogenated or partially hydrogenated oils, Shortening, Deep-fried foods, Crackers (most), Cookies (most), Mayonnaise, Potato chips, Breakfast cereal (most), Cake and muffin mixes (most)

SATURATED FATS

Saturated fats are those fats that are solid at room temperature, including butterfat, most animal fats, and coconut, palm, and palm kernel oils. Saturated fats either are used for energy or are stored as body fat for future use. The bad news about saturated fats is that they tend to raise the level of cholesterol and fat in the blood, both of which increase the risk of heart disease. Your body can make saturated fat from other fats, so you really don't need to consume saturated fat at all. But meat and dairy products are a mainstay of our diet and include some of our favorite foods, such as ice cream and hamburgers. Common sense dictates that saturated fat should be consumed in moderation, generally limited to a *maxium* of 10 percent of your daily calories, which equals about 20 to 25 grams per day, depending on your size. (Food labeling laws now require that the saturated fat content of packaged foods be listed as a separate category, making it relatively easy to track your intake.)

TRANS FATS

Trans fats are a man-made type of fat, created when unsaturated fats are artificially saturated through a process called hydrogenation. In their natural state, fatty acids are fashioned in a three-dimensional configuration called a cis-form. By applying heat and special catalysts, the hydrogenation process rearranges the molecules to a different shape called the trans-form. The resulting fatty acids are known as *trans fatty acids*.

Hydrogenation turns an oil that normally would be liquid at room temperature into a fat that is solid at room temperature. Pick up any package of cookies, crackers, cereals—almost any packaged food you can think of—and most likely you will see partially hydrogenated oils listed in the ingredients. By some estimates, we eat twenty-five times as much hydrogenated fat today as we did seventy-five years ago. Food manufacturers love hydrogenated fats because they are far more stable than the natural forms of the oils, giving these products extended shelf life.

Although they are technically unsaturated fats, trans fats behave like saturated fats in that they raise your LDL cholesterol (the "bad" cholesterol). In fact, several studies show that hydrogenated fats are even more dangerous than saturated fats because they also lower your HDL (or "good") cholesterol. In addition, hydrogenated oils may increase your risk of breast cancer and interfere with detoxification of the liver. It has been estimated that trans fats are responsible for 30,000 deaths a year in the United States, chiefly through their dangerous effect on cholesterol levels.

Unfortunately, food manufacturers are not required to list the amount of trans fats in a product, which can make it difficult to know how much of the dangerous fat you may be consuming. Today most people eat from 5 to 10 percent of their total calories as trans fats. Anything over 5 percent is considered to be dangerous to good health, but obviously no amount can be considered healthy.

MONOUNSATURATED FATS

These are the fats that are liquid at room temperature but solid or semisolid when refrigerated. The most well-known sources of monounsaturated fats are olive and canola oil. (Avocados are also high in monounsaturated fats.)

Monounsaturated fats are known for their heart-healthy benefits, lowering bad cholesterol and helping to decrease oxidation of cholesterol in the blood vessels. The body can manufacture monounsaturated fats from other fats in the diet, so they are not technically essential for good health. However, a big advantage of the monounsaturated fats is that they are very stable and don't spoil, or oxidize, as easily as other fats.

The most dangerous fat of all is an oxidized fat. When fats oxidize, either inside or outside the body, they create large quantities of free radical molecules. These highly reactive molecules are a major cause of the cellular damage that can lead to cancer, heart disease, and other diseases. Buying small quantities of oil and keeping them away from heat and light will help minimize this health risk. Using olive and canola oil instead of more unstable oils is also a healthful choice. Never use any oil or fat that has a sour or rancid smell.

Monounsaturated oils also are the only fats that are not associated with an increase in disease, even when they make up quite a high percentage of daily calories. By comparison, a high intake of saturated fats is associated with an increased risk of heart disease. Similarly, high intakes of polyunsaturated fats (discussed later) have been linked to a higher incidence of cancer. For all of these reasons, monounsaturated fats should comprise the majority of your daily fat intake, up to 15 to 20 percent of daily calorie intake.

POLYUNSATURATED FATS

You can tell a polyunsaturated fat because it will remain liquid even when refrigerated. Most common vegetable oils, such as corn, safflower, sunflower, peanut, cottonseed, and soybean, are high in polyunsaturated fats. Also included in the polyunsaturated family are some less common oils, such as sesame, flax, borage, grapeseed, and evening primrose oil.

Polyunsaturated fats tend to be rather unstable and oxidize quite easily. As noted earlier, oxidized oils are a potent source of free radicals, which can do extensive cellular damage. Oxidative damage is implicated in almost every degenerative disease but is particularly associated with cancer. Most polyunsaturated fats contain small amounts of vitamin E as a natural antioxidant and preservative. Nonetheless, they need to be handled carefully to protect them from degradation.

Polyunsaturated fats are extremely important to health because they are the only source of *essential fatty acids*, those fatty acids that cannot be manufactured by the body, and *must* be gotten from the diet. Unlike other types of fat, EFAs are not generally burned for energy or stored as fat but instead are used in countless biochemical operations throughout the body. In order to ensure adequate intake of EFAs, 5 to 10 percent of your daily fat intake should be essential fatty acids from polyunsaturated fats.

ESSENTIAL FATTY ACIDS

There is some controversy in the scientific community as to which fatty acids are truly essential. The most widely accepted view is that there are two essential fatty acids, alpha-linolenic acid (ALA) and linoleic acid (LA). Oils high in ALA, including those from fish, flax, canola, and walnuts, are called omega-3 oils. (We'll talk more about the omega-3 family of fats in Chapter 6.) Oils that contain a lot of linoleic acid often are referred to as omega-6 oils. These include some of the most common commercial cooking oils, such as those made from corn, safflowers, sunflowers, soybeans, peanuts, and sesame seeds. Evening primrose oil also belongs to the omega-6 family, but it is a special case because, in addition to linoleic acid, it is also a rich source of the more rarely found GLA.

By the strictest definition, however, a nutrient is considered essential only when it *cannot* be manufactured within the body and *must* be consumed in the diet. By this definition, linoleic acid is the only essential fatty acid, since the body can manufacture ALA from LA, but not the reverse.

Note: Polyunsaturated oils that have been artificially hydrogenated no longer contain any essential fatty acids, so hydrogenated oils, even if they are made from polyunsaturated oils, belong to the trans fat category.

In addition to being somewhat controversial, the

term "essential fatty acid," is also somewhat mis-leading because, before they can really do any good in the body, EFAs first must be converted to other compounds. Linoleic acid, for example, is ineffective in the body until it has been converted to another, more active fatty acid called gamma-linolenic acid (GLA). Similarly, alpha-linolenic acid must be converted in the body to eicosapentaenoic acid (EPA) and docosahexaenoic acid (DHA).

Although LA and sometimes ALA are considered to be *essential* fatty acids, the three most *important* fatty acids for human health are EPA, DHA, and GLA. If these three are not present in the diet, and if the body, for one reason or another, cannot manufacture them from other raw materials, the body will likely show signs of fatty acid deficiencies, no matter how much fat is being consumed.

Fatty Acid Deficiency

It may be hard to imagine that you could be suffering from a fat deficiency. After all, for years you've been told that you are eating too much fat. However, if you are not getting the particular fatty acids you need, or if your body is not making them for you, you will almost certainly display symptoms of essential fatty acid deficiency. Scientists estimate that, for optimal health, we should consume a minimum of 7 to 10 grams of EFAs each day, but most of us fall far short of this mark.

Signs of fatty acid deficiency include:

- *Hair loss*
- *Painful swollen joints*
- *Dry, scaly skin*
- *Weak, brittle nails*
- *Acne*
- *Eczema*
- *Infertility*
- *Dry eyes*
- *Dry mouth*
- *Circulatory problems*
- *Poor wound healing*

BEYOND EFAS

Your body converts EFAs to more active compounds in a series of steps that involve various enzymatic reactions. In the case of linoleic acid, the first step is its conversion to gamma-linolenic acid, which requires an enzyme called delta-6-desaturase. As we already know, GLA is an extremely crucial nutrient for good health, but, again, it is only a stepping-stone. It, in turn, goes through several more metabolic steps, being converted further into dihomo-gamma-linolenic acid (DGLA) and finally into very potent molecules known as prostaglandins.

PROSTAGLANDINS

Prostaglandins are hormonelike compounds that control hundreds of important functions in the body. These potent chemicals, discovered only in

Figure 2.1. Essential Fatty Acid Pathway

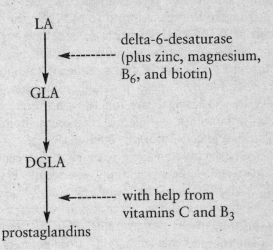

the 1970s, play a role in regulating blood pressure, blood clotting, cholesterol levels, inflammation, allergic reactivity, hormone activity, immune function, neurological function, and more.

Preformed prostaglandins are not readily available in our food supply and most likely would be destroyed by the digestive process even if they were. Instead, the body manufactures prostaglandins throughout the body as needed, using fatty acids as building blocks. Once created, prostaglandins have only a short time to perform their designated functions before they are quickly deactivated by enzymes. Because they are so short lived, it is important to have a ready and constant supply of fatty acids with which to fuel pros-taglandin synthesis.

There are dozens of different prostaglandins,

which are divided into families designated by letters of the alphabet. (For example, the "A" family of prostaglandins are referred to as PGAs, the "B" family as PGBs, etc.) Scientists are still figuring out how the various prostaglandins function, but one of the most interesting and significant families is the PGE family. These prostaglandins are very active in regulating heart function, hormone balance, inflammation, allergic response, immune function, and certain brain functions.

Most of the prostaglandin research to date centers on members of the PGE family, specifically PGE1, PGE2, and PGE3. The numbers simply denote which fatty acid is the parent molecule of that particular prostaglandin. For example, PGE1 is derived from gamma-linolenic acid, PGE2 from arachidonic acid (AA), and PGE3 from eicosapentaenoic acid.

If you have read anything about prostaglandins, you may have seen PGE1 and PGE3 referred to as "good" prostaglandins and PGE2 as the "bad" prostaglandin. The so-called good prostaglandins have a number of beneficial effects, such as reducing inflammation and blood clotting and lowering blood pressure and cholesterol, while PGE2 acts in opposition to the other two, tending to increase inflammation, blood pressure, and blood stickiness.

It is important to keep in mind, however, that the actions of PGE2 are, under certain circumstances, both necessary and beneficial. The various prostaglandins are designed to work in concert, with opposing actions that serve as checks and bal-

Figure 2.2. The Prostaglandin Pathways

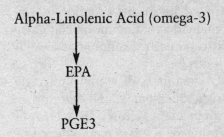

Alpha-Linolenic Acid (omega-3)

EPA

PGE3

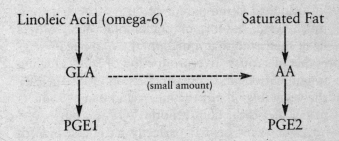

Linoleic Acid (omega-6)   Saturated Fat

GLA - - - - - - - - - - - - - - - - - -> AA
          (small amount)

PGE1   PGE2

ances to keep the body in equilibrium. While PGE1
and PGE3 keep the blood pressure from getting
dangerously high, for example, PGE2 ensures that
blood pressure doesn't dip too low.

A WORD ABOUT ARACHIDONIC ACID
Many health conditions, such as arthritis, premenstrual syndrome, cardiovascular disease, allergies,
and immune disorders, are linked to overactivity of
PGE2 prostaglandins, which tend to cause inflam-

mation, raise blood pressure, and fuel allergic reactions. As the precursor of PGE2, arachidonic acid often is seen as the villain in this situation. Many nutritionists recommend avoiding meats and dairy products in order to reduce the amount of arachidonic acid in the body.

Most of the AA in our bodies comes directly from dietary sources, chiefly meat and dairy products, but it also can be manufactured from GLA in the body. This is not a very active metabolic pathway, however, and accounts for only a small percentage of the AA supply. Nonetheless, because linoleic acid is the parent of both GLA and, to a much lesser extent, of arachidonic acid, others have suggested that a high intake of omega-6 vegetable oils causes overproduction of PGE2, fueling inflammation and disease. But, in truth, neither the vegetable oil nor the meats and dairy products in our diet is the culprit in the PGE2 scenario.

Arachidonic acid is perfectly harmless; indeed, it's absolutely necessary for good health. The level of PGE1 in our cells regulates the amount of PGE2 prostaglandins that are produced from arachidonic acid. As long as our bodies are producing plenty of PGE1, the conversion of arachidonic acid into PGE2 is held strictly in check. However, in the absence of sufficient PGE1, the conversion of arachidonic acid into PGE2 is greatly enhanced. In short, science has shown that the most effective way to keep PGE2 production under control is to enhance production of PGE1 with essential fatty acid precursors like evening primrose oil.

Figure 2.3. Prostaglandin Checks and Balances

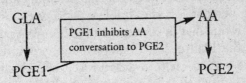

There's no doubt that many of today's health problems are caused (or at least accompanied) by excessive PGE2 production. But, as we have seen, this is less likely to be the result of too much arachidonic acid in the diet and more likely to be an indication of low levels of PGE1 prostaglandins. And yet the parent molecule of PGE1, linoleic acid, is very plentiful in our diets, accounting for approximately 10 to 12 percent of our daily calorie intake. According to everything we've seen so far, we should be producing more than enough PGE1 prostaglandins! And yet modern health statistics suggest that deficiency of PGE1 is widespread. So what's the problem?

THE MISSING LINK

The metabolic pathway that leads to the production of PGE1 prostaglandins begins with linoleic acid, a fatty acid that is plentiful in our diets. Most of us consume somewhere in the range of 20 to 25 grams a day of this type of fat. However, several things can block the very first step on this path, namely, the conversion of linoleic acid to GLA. Even under the best of circumstances, only about 5 to 10 percent of the linoleic acid we take in through our diet is converted to GLA. As you can see in the Figure 2.1, this conversion requires an enzyme called delta-6-desaturase, of which we have a limited supply. The amount of GLA we can produce is limited to the amount of this enzyme available. The rest of the linoleic acid we eat is used to maintain cell membranes and for other structural purposes throughout the body.

Many people are born with an inability to produce this enzyme, and can manufacture only a very small amount of GLA or none at all. For these people, the metabolic chain that leads to the production of beneficial prostaglandins never gets beyond the very first step. As we'll see in later chapters, this genetic anomaly appears to be a factor in some inherited illnesses. In addition to delta-6-desaturase, the conversion of linoleic acid requires several other nutrients, including B_6, zinc, magnesium, calcium, and vitamin C. Low levels of any of these important nutrients can hinder the metabolic process that produces both GLA and PGE1.

Many other lifestyle and environmental factors can block the conversion of linoleic acid, including alcohol consumption, diabetes, cancer, stress, high cholesterol, and viral infections. Even the normal aging process appears to hinder our ability to manufacture GLA and PGE1.

As you can see, the metabolic path from linoleic

Figure 2.4. Upsetting the Balance: Lifestyle Considerations

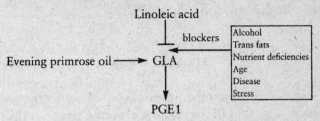

acid to PGE1 is strewn with roadblocks, but perhaps the biggest culprits are those relative new-
comers, the trans fatty acids. As our consumption
of trans fatty acids has increased, the signs of
essential fatty acid deficiency have become increasingly evident. More and more of the fat we eat is
biologically inactive in our bodies and is actually
preventing the good fats from getting the job done.

These artificially created trans fatty acids are so
similar in shape to the naturally occurring forms of
the fatty acids that they can take their place in cell
membranes. But although the trans fatty acid fits
into the keyhole, it won't turn the lock. Trans fats
are unable to carry out any of the metabolic
processes of natural fatty acids, including conversion to prostaglandins. Trans fats actually increase
the body's requirement for essential fatty acids.
The more trans fats you eat, the more essential
fatty acids you need to compensate.

But if the body, for any one of the reasons listed
here, can't convert linoleic acid to GLA, it doesn't

matter how much linoleic acid is present in the diet: The manufacture of PGE1 will be hindered, and health will suffer as a result.

THE SOLUTION

Here's where evening primrose oil comes into our story. The seed of the evening primrose is one of the vegetable kingdom's richest sources of naturally occurring GLA. By supplying gamma-linolenic acid, evening primrose oil bypasses the many pitfalls that block the conversion of linoleic acid. With a ready supply of active GLA, the body can resume production of beneficial prostaglandins, correcting most of the symptoms of EFA deficiency in short order.

Evening primrose oil contains anywhere from 8.8 to 10.5 percent GLA. The balance of the oil is mostly linoleic acid, with a small percentage of other fatty acids.

Typical Composition of Evening Primrose oil
Linoleic Acid (LA): 74.6%
Gamma-linolenic Acid (GLA): 9.1%
Oleic Acid (a non-essential fatty acid): 9.0%
Saturated fatty acids: 7.3%

As a supplement, evening primrose is most frequently packaged in gel capsules, each of which contains 500 milligrams (mg) of the oil, providing approximately 45 mg GLA. For general nutritional support, three capsules per day will help to rebalance fatty acid profiles and optimize prostaglandin production. In the treatment of serious imbalances or deficiencies, evening primrose can be taken in much higher quantities, up to 20 capsules, or 10 grams, a day, without problems.

As you will learn in the following chapters, evening primrose oil can be used in the treatment of allergies, asthma, arthritis, PMS, high cholesterol and blood pressure, diabetes, autoimmune disease, and many other health conditions. It also can help you lose weight, keep your skin clear, and make your nails and hair strong.

OTHER SOURCES

Since the discovery of evening primrose oil as a source of gammalinolenic acid, a few other natural sources of GLA have been discovered, including borage seed oil and black currant seed oil. In each of these, the percentage of GLA is actually significantly higher than in evening primrose. Borage seed oil is approximately 22 to 24 percent GLA. Perhaps not coincidentally, borage was used in the Middle Ages as a herbal remedy for inflammation, heart disease, and rheumatism. Oil pressed from the seeds of blackcurrants also has been discovered to contain high amounts of GLA—about 18 to 20 percent. Both borage seed oil and black currant seed oil are being marketed as alternatives to evening primrose oil. Because of the higher percentage of GLA in these oils, they claim to be more cost-effective, delivering the same amount of GLA in fewer capsules.

The therapeutic actions of evening primrose oil are clearly due to its GLA content, and so it is reasonable to expect that other sources of GLA would offer the same benefits. However, research comparing the biological activity of the different sources of GLA has indicated otherwise. When measured by changes in fatty acid profiles and prostaglandin activity, evening primrose oil appears to be much more biologically active than either borage or black currant seed oil, even though these other oils contain a higher percentage of GLA.

When scientists analyze healing plants and other natural substances, they often attempt to identify and isolate a single active component responsible for the effect. But nature frequently designs subtle and complex delivery systems for natural medicines that cannot be reduced to a single chemical agent. Apparently, the particular makeup of evening primrose, including the exact combination and amounts of other fatty acids present in the oil, has something to do with its effectiveness. Any cost savings that might be afforded by the use of borage or black currant seed oil as a source of GLA evaporates if one has to take greater quantities to get the same effect as evening primrose oil provides.

Now, on to the specifics of using evening primrose oil for maximum health, wellness, and beauty.

3

A Solution for Premenstrual Syndrome

YOU'VE probably heard more than a few jokes about PMS . . . featuring chocolate-crazed women stealing candy from the children's Halloween stash, bursting into tears over misplaced car keys, or subjecting hapless mates to unprovoked outbursts of irrational fury. While keeping a sense of humor never hurts, if you are one of the 30 million American women who suffer from this chronic condition, you know that premenstrual syndrome (PMS) is no joke. It's a serious medical condition that can steal days and weeks out of every month, at the expense of jobs, families, and personal time.

Even during these times of incredible medical advancement and sophistication, PMS continues to frustrate both those who suffer from it and those who aim to ease that suffering. Exactly what causes this vexing condition has proven to be an elusive and much-debated question. Unable to find (or agree on) the smoking gun, conventional medical treatment for PMS has been limited to stamping out the symptomatic brushfires with a variety of drugs, discussed later in this chapter.

Fortunately, nature has provided a wonderfully effective remedy for premenstrual syndrome in the form of evening primrose oil. This marvelous natural substance brings rapid, drug-free relief for most PMS symptoms, simply by rebalancing the body's essential fatty acid biochemistry. Numerous scientific studies confirm what hundreds of thousands of women already know from personal experience—that adding evening primrose oil to your diet can make this monthly misery a thing of the past.

WHAT EXACTLY IS PMS?

Almost every woman experiences one or more premenstrual symptoms at some point in her life. But when the symptoms begin to interfere with everyday activities, it is considered to be premenstrual syndrome. Many women don't see a doctor about PMS symptoms, so it is hard to say for sure how common the syndrome is. Estimates can vary widely, but most experts agree that about four in ten women between the ages of fifteen and fifty-five are affected by PMS. It is even more commonly reported in women between the ages of thirty and forty, affecting about six in ten. Of all women with PMS, about 10 percent have severe forms of the condition.

PMS RISK FACTORS

PMS is reported more often by women who:

- Have had children
- Had complications such as toxemia during pregnancy
- Tend to experience menstrual pain and cramping
- Do not exercise regularly
- Have high stress levels
- Consume high amounts of salt and/or sugar

All in all, over 150 different symptoms, including physical, mental, and/or emotional changes, have been attributed to PMS. The most common physical symptoms include:

- Bloating and weight gain
- Painful breasts
- Headaches
- Back pain
- Acne
- Hives
- Joint pain
- Constipation

Mood disturbances and mental changes related to PMS include:

- Mood swings
- Depression
- Irritability
- Fatigue
- Anxiety or nervousness
- Difficulty in concentrating
- Memory loss
- Cravings for sweets and carbohydrates

Symptoms typically begin anywhere from several days to two weeks prior to menstruation and usually stop soon after the period begins. They range in severity from unpleasant to utterly debilitating, even leading women to suicide in extreme cases.

Are You Suffering from PMS?

There is no laboratory test for PMS. Usually it is diagnosed based on a patient's report of her symptoms. Many doctors ask their patients to keep a symptom diary for two or three menstrual cycles, which can serve not only as a diagnostic tool but also as a way of monitoring the effectiveness of treatment.

To make your own chart, begin on the first day of your period. Each day, note any symptoms you are feeling (headache, breast tenderness, irritability, changes in appetite, etc.) and the degree of severity (1 for severe, 2 for moderate, and 3 for mild). Keep your diary for several complete menstrual cycles.

When evaluating your chart, ask yourself the following questions:

- Do your symptoms occur more frequently or increase in severity during the two weeks before your period?
- Do your symptoms quickly diminish when your period begins?
- Do your symptoms interfere with your ability to work, exercise, or perform other daily activities?

If you answer yes to all of these questions, you are most likely suffering from premenstrual syndrome.

As if the reality of PMS were not bad enough, up until quite recently it was commonly dismissed as the product of an overwrought female imagination, possibly because of the less tangible, emotional aspect of many of the symptoms. Perhaps this attitude has its roots in the ancient Greek writings that still influence our modern medical culture.

For example, the word "hysteria" stems from the Greek word for uterus (*hystera*), reflecting the once widely held belief that the mere presence of a uterus predisposed females to emotional or mental instability. In fact, hysterectomies were routinely performed in the 19th century as a cure for "excessive" emotionality or sexual "dysfunctions" such as excessive libido.

It wasn't until the twentieth century that scientists came to recognize the existence of the different sex hormones and how they affect men's and women's health. We've also come to understand that psychological symptoms are often purely biochemical, caused by imbalances of brain chemicals called *neurotransmitters*. Only very recently did premenstrual syndrome achieve recognition as a legitimate medical condition.

Nonetheless, medical "treatment" for PMS remains relatively primitive, consisting of various drugs that simply mask the symptoms rather than getting at the root of the problem.

COMMON MEDICAL TREATMENTS FOR PMS

PAIN RELIEVERS

Ibuprofen and acetaminophen are commonly prescribed for PMS-related discomforts and frequently show up in over-the-counter PMS preparations as well. These drugs are often effective in relieving headaches, backaches, and joint pain associated with PMS, but they are not without drawbacks, especially when used frequently or over long periods of time.

Ibuprofen (Motrin, Advil, Nuprin) belongs to a class of pain relievers known as nonsteroidal anti-inflammatories, or NSAIDs. These are extremely irritating to the digestive tract and can cause pain, ulcers, and bleeding in the stomach. (Frequent use of NSAIDs eventually can lead to anemia, due to blood loss from the stomach.) Ironically, excess fluid retention is one of the side effects of ibuprofen.

Because it is gentler on the stomach, acetaminophen (Tylenol) is often considered to be a safer pain reliever. But acetaminophen puts a significant strain on the liver, depleting its reserves of glutathione, one of the body's most critical detoxifying nutrients. In fact, acetaminophen poisoning is one of the most severe types and can lead to liver failure in a matter of hours. When combined with even moderate amounts of alcohol, even normal acetaminophen usage can cause serious liver damage.

DIURETICS

Because many of the symptoms of PMS are due to excessive water retention, many women turn to diuretics, or "water pills." These can provide temporary symptom relief, but diuretics can leach important minerals from the body, especially potassium and magnesium. Potassium deficiency also can lead to depression and, of all things, PMS. Natural diuretics such as dandelion or other herbs (available in capsules or teas, also can lead to potassium and other mineral deficiencies, if overused.

A newer diuretic called spironolactone (Alatone, Aldactone, Novospiroton, Spironazide) has a mild diuretic effect without causing excess potassium loss, and often it is used in combination with other diuretics to prevent depletion of the body's potassium reserves. However, it carries the risk of masculinizing effects, such as excessive hair growth and deepening of the voice. It also can cause hepatitis and liver damage.

ANTIDEPRESSANTS

When PMS is accompanied by significant depression or other mood disturbances, it may be treated with antidepressant medications like Prozac, Zoloft, or Paxil. These drugs are selective serotonin reuptake inhibitors (SSRIs), acting to increase the amount of serotonin in the brain.

Women who suffer from PMS often have abnormally low levels of serotonin, an important neurotransmitter that affects mood, appetite, and other functions including digestion, sleep, pain sensitivity, and body temperature. Many times raising these levels with antidepressant medications can ease some of the mood-related symptoms of PMS, but nearly 20 percent of people find the side effects so unpleasant that they discontinue taking the drugs. Common adverse reactions include nausea, headaches, insomnia, drowsiness, and impaired sexual function (for both men and women).

In addition, people often find that antidepressants dull both the "ups" and the "downs" and leave them feeling uncomfortably flat and emotionally detached. For many women, these drawbacks outweigh the benefits. In Chapter 4 you'll learn about natural alternatives that can rebalance serotonin levels without these side effects.

OTHER DRUGS

When patients don't get relief from these relatively conservative approaches, doctors sometimes resort to more drastic pharmaceutical interventions, including antianxiety medications (which can be addictive), birth control pills, or even hormones that bring on chemically induced menopause.

While they sometimes provide temporary relief, each of these drugs comes with its own set of risks and side effects, and none addresses the true cause of the problem. Eliminating the menstrual cycle with artificial hormones is, after all, a relatively extreme solution. It's important to remember that menstruation, with its attendant hormonal fluctuations, is not a disease or illness but a normal, healthy occurrence. When there are problems related to the menstrual cycle—such as PMS, severe menstrual cramps, or abnormally heavy bleeding—it is a signal that the body's natural balance has been disturbed.

GETTING TO THE ROOT OF THE PROBLEM

It is largely the presence (or lack) of essential fatty acids in your body, especially the gamma-linolenic acid (GLA) found in evening primrose oil, that determines whether you sail through your monthly cycle without a problem or suffer the discomforts of PMS.

Researchers studying premenstrual syndrome have found that women with PMS tend to be particularly low in essential fatty acids. At St. Thomas Hospital in London, Dr. Michael Brush conducted a study of sixty-five women with moderate to severe PMS, all of whom had tried one or more of the standard medical treatments for PMS, without success. For the study, the subjects increased their intake of essential fatty acids by taking evening primrose oil capsules (two to three 500-mg capsules, twice a day). The results were quite impressive. Nearly two-thirds of the women in the study (61 percent) reported *complete relief* from PMS symptoms, including mood swings, anxiety, irritability, headaches, water retention, and painful breasts. An additional 23 percent reported partial relief.

Several other studies, including double-blind, placebo-controlled trials conducted at research centers around Europe, have confirmed that evening primrose oil is highly effective in relieving symptoms of PMS. In every study, improvements were seen after only one month of treatment, and longer-term studies showed that symptoms continued to improve for up to five months. The relief lasted as long as women continued taking evening primrose oil, and the symptoms tended to return if it was discontinued. From the research conducted to date, the dosage that appears most effective is six to eight capsules (500 mg each) per day.

It may be hard to believe that something as complex as PMS could be tamed through the simple addition of a teaspoon or so of a natural plant extract. (And PMS is just one of many serious health conditions that this amazing food benefits.) How does evening primrose oil work these many miracles?

PMS AND PROSTAGLANDINS

As we saw in Chapter 2, evening primrose oil supports your body's production of important hormonelike compounds called prostaglandins. And these prostaglandins, in turn, have a direct impact on the symptoms of premenstrual syndrome.

Specifically, evening primrose oil supplies the precursors that your body needs in order to manufacture PGE1. One of the so-called "good" prostaglandins, PGE1 is a natural anti-inflammatory and anti-spasmodic agent, helping to prevent back and joint pain often associated with PMS. It is also a natural diuretic, preventing fluid buildup that can cause temporary weight gain, bloating, breast tenderness, headaches, and irritability. Not surprisingly, women with PMS tend to have particularly low levels of PGE1.

BALANCE IS EVERYTHING

One important function of PGE1 is to offset the effects of PGE2, sometimes referred to as the "bad" prostaglandin because it promotes inflam-

mation and fluid retention. This good guy/bad guy
view of prostaglandins is, of course, an oversimplification. In certain circumstances, such as injury or
infection, inflammation serves a valuable healing
and protective function. But if the body can't make
enough PGE1 to balance the inflammatory tendencies of PGE2, excessive water retention and inflammation can translate into troublesome—and
unnecessary—back and joint pain, headaches,
breast tenderness, and other PMS symptoms.

Many women reach for over-the-counter pain
relievers like Motrin or Advil when PMS symptoms strike. These nonsteroidal anti-inflammatory
drugs ease pain and inflammation by blocking the
production of inflammatory PGE2. Unfortunately,
they also block production of beneficial PGE1, and
they can damage your stomach and kidneys with
prolonged use.

Evening primrose oil is a more natural solution
for PMS discomforts, supplying the essential fatty
acids that your body uses to make PGE1. By
shifting prostaglandin production away from the
pro-inflammatory PGE2 and toward the anti-
inflammatory PGE1, evening primrose oil naturally eases PMS symptoms without side effects.

THE EMOTIONAL ASPECT OF PMS

Women using evening primrose oil also notice significant improvement in the emotional symptoms

of PMS, such as intense mood swings, depression, anxiety, and irritability. In our earlier discussion of conventional medical treatments for PMS, we saw that women with this condition often have low serotonin levels. Although the relationships are not fully understood, prostaglandins do play a role in the body's production of serotonin and other neurotransmitters, which may explain how evening primrose oil regulates emotional and mood-related symptoms.

PGE1 also seems to affect the way the body responds to *prolactin*, a hormone that stimulates milk production. Pregnant women and nursing mothers generate high levels of prolactin, but all women produce it in small amounts. In addition to triggering the production of breast milk, high prolactin levels also are thought to play a part in the extreme emotional volatility many women experience during and after pregnancy.

When researchers noticed that injections of prolactin bring on fluid retention, irritability, and other PMS-like symptoms in male subjects, they investigated the connection further to see if PMS symptoms could be caused in part by an excess of prolactin. They found instead that women with premenstrual syndrome do *not* have elevated levels of the hormone. However, some scientists now suspect that the lack of PGE1 prostaglandins, which *is* common to women with PMS, may cause a hypersensitivity to prolactin's effects. Enhancing PGE1 levels with evening primrose oil appears to reverse

this oversensitivity and may partly explain its
effectiveness in reducing both physical and emotional symptoms of PMS.

EVENING PRIMROSE OIL:
MAKING A DIFFERENCE

Joanne is a trial lawyer for the state's attorney's
office. Although she always makes an effort to present a polished, professional appearance in court,
premenstrual water retention and bloating made her
tailored, size-10 suits too tight to wear for a week or
more out of every month. At considerable expense,
Joanne ended up investing in two suit wardrobes—
one in her "normal" size and another in her "PMS"
size. She also noticed that she had difficulty concentrating and was not as sharp in court during her premenstrual phase. With little control over the
scheduling of her cases, she often worried about the
way it affected her job performance.

On the advice of a coworker, Joanne began taking evening primrose oil twice a day and noticed a
difference in only a few weeks. She no longer bal-
looned to a larger dress size before her period—in
fact, to her amazement, she lost four pounds
without changing her diet. She also noticed that
she didn't seem to get that fuzzy, unfocused feeling before her period. Joanne donated her size-12
suits to a women's shelter and vowed to make
evening primrose oil a lifetime habit.

* * *

Kim, an enthusiastic runner who logged three or four miles a day, usually had to stop running during the week or so before her period, because of tender, painful breasts and sore joints. More than once she was forced to withdraw at the last minute from races and other events that she had trained for and looked forward to, because they fell during her premenstrual week. Although she often felt depressed over the extent to which PMS interfered with her life, Kim assumed that it was simply "in her genes," because both of her sisters suffered symptoms as well.

Kim found that evening primrose oil supplements virtually eliminated the breast tenderness and joint pain she'd experienced and allowed her to maintain her daily running regimen right through her monthly cycle. She also noticed that she had to use her asthma inhaler much less often when exercising, which made running even more pleasant. Within six months of starting evening primrose oil, Kim trained for and completed her first half-marathon race. She also recommended evening primrose to her sisters as a solution for their monthly battles with PMS symptoms.

* * *

Felice lost her job as an executive secretary because severe PMS symptoms caused her to call in sick too often. She spent three or four days each month battling severe headaches, back pain, and an overwhelming cloud of depression and lethargy that made it difficult to get out of bed, much less function effectively at work. Over-the-counter pain relievers did little to relieve her aching head and back, and Felice often resorted to sleeping aids to get through the dreaded monthly attacks. She was too embarrassed to tell anyone why she lost her job and was afraid to use her employer as a reference for a new position.

After losing her job, Felice struggled with feelings of depression and hopelessness for several months. She finally sought help from a nutrition-oriented physician, who put her on a regimen of dietary supplements that included evening primrose oil and helped her make gradual but significant changes in her diet. (See Chapter 4 for your own complete PMS prevention plan.)

Felice felt a difference within the first month, and after four months she reported that she no longer had any significant symptoms whatsoever. Feeling as if she'd been given a brand-new start in life, Felice decided to make a career change and returned to school to study nutrition and herbology. She is planning a career as a nutrition and wellness counselor, teaching women how to take charge of their health with nutrition and natural therapies.

A WORD ABOUT FIBROCYSTIC (BENIGN) BREAST DISEASE

In many of the studies discussed already, researchers noted that evening primrose oil is especially effective in treating cyclical breast pain (soreness and tenderness that comes and goes throughout the monthly cycle). Several clinics devoted exclusively to breast health have extended this research into the treatment of other breast disorders with evening primrose oil.

About 30 to 40 percent of women are affected by significant breast pain or tenderness (mastalgia), which may or may not be accompanied by painful, noncancerous lumps in the breast (also known as fibrocystic breast disease). In the vast majority of cases, the symptoms are cyclical, increasing during the premenstrual phase and resolving or improving when menstruation begins. In the case of fibrocystic breast disease, the physical discomfort can be compounded by emotional anguish aroused by the fear that the lumps could be cancerous.

Researchers analyzed thirty-two different clinical studies on women with breast pain and ranked evening primrose oil in the highest category of effectiveness. Doctors at the Cardiff Mastalgia Clinic in Wales, a center that focuses solely on the treatment of severe breast pain, recently did a case review of 414 patients treated at the clinic over a seventeen-year period. They found that evening primrose oil was as effective in relieving breast pain as drugs that are commonly used to treat this condition—only with far fewer side effects.

DRUGS USED TO TREAT SEVERE BREAST PAIN

When the severity of breast pain causes a significant disruption of normal activities, doctors may prescribe several drugs. The one thing that all the drugs have in common is that they reduce the levels of prolactin, a hormone that can cause breast pain, swelling, and tenderness.

Danazol is a drug derived from testosterone that reduces the levels of estrogen and prolactin in the blood and increases levels of circulating testosterone. Danazol also prevents ovulation, which may or may not be desirable, and has a detrimental effect on cholesterol ratios. It is effective in reducing cyclical breast pain but has a high rate of adverse reactions. The Cardiff Mastalgia Clinic reports that fully one-third of women treated with danazol complained of significant side effects, the most common of which were weight gain, menstrual irregularity, headaches, nausea, and acne. Less common were depression, reduced breast size, hair loss, excessive facial hair, and a deepened voice. (These masculinizing effects are common to drugs that raise testosterone levels in women.) About one sixth of the women stopped the treatment, even when it was successful in relieving symptoms, because the side effects were intolerable.

Bromocriptine reduces prolactin levels by suppressing its release from the pituitary gland but does not affect testosterone or estrogen levels. Originally developed for the treatment of Parkinson's disease, it is less effective than danazol in relieving breast pain but has an even higher incidence of side effects. Although bromocriptine doesn't have the sort of masculinizing effects seen with danazol, one in five of the women studied experienced nausea and vomiting, and one tenth suffered headaches. Other side effects included constipation, indigestion, and depression. Ultimately, about one fifth of the women studied opted to stop using the drug.

A NATURAL TREATMENT FOR BREAST PAIN

Evening primrose oil is an excellent alternative to high-risk drug therapies for breast pain. By decreasing sensitivity to prolactin, it is highly effective in relieving symptoms and is virtually free of side effects. The Cardiff Mastalgia Clinic reports that only 4 percent of the women treated with evening primrose oil complained of side effects, which included nausea, headache, depression, and rash. Only one in fifty patients decided to discontinue treatment.

The dose used for benign breast disease is similar to that found to be effective for premenstrual syndrome—between six and eight capsules (500 mg each) per day. (Complete protocols and dosage recommendations for premenstrual syndrome and other menstrual disorders are detailed in Chapter 4.) Doctors who recommend evening primrose are careful to explain to their patients that symptoms improve gradually; although many women notice a difference right away, it can take several months for the benefits to become fully apparent. In general, the longer women continue treatment, the better the results. In some cases, symptoms began to respond after a month or two and then continued to improve for up to twelve months.

Fortunately, evening primrose oil is a safe and relatively inexpensive therapy that also has a multitude of other health benefits, making it all the more attractive to continue indefinitely.

OTHER MENSTRUAL IRREGULARITIES

Menstrual cramps affect over half of all menstruating women. Again, the culprit may be an overabundance of PGE2, which is not only pro-inflammatory but also encourages muscle spasms. When the muscles of the uterus contract, the resulting lack of oxygen causes painful uterine cramps.

An effective way to prevent menstrual cramps is to increase production of PGE1 prostaglandins, the body's natural antispasmodic compounds. The addition of evening primrose oil supplements can frequently reduce or eliminate menstrual cramps.

Excessive bleeding during menstruation is not only a nuisance but eventually can lead to anemia if the iron lost via the menstrual flow is not replaced through iron-rich foods or iron supplements. NSAIDs such as ibuprofen can reduce menstrual flow by blocking production of PGE2, but a more natural way to get the same effect is to boost the levels of anti-inflammatory PGE1, which also dampens the effect of the inflammatory PGE2. Once again, evening primrose oil supplements can be very helpful, reducing heavy bleeding as well as the need for harsh anti-inflammatory drugs.

SUMMING UP THE EVIDENCE

With our increasing reliance on highly processed, prepackaged convenience foods, our modern diet has become dangerously deficient in essential fatty acids and other nutrients necessary for proper EFA metabolism. Although commonly overlooked, this nutritional shortfall appears to be a culprit in the growing incidence and severity of PMS as well as many other health conditions discussed throughout this book.

A wealth of scientific research shows that evening primrose oil fills this critical nutritional gap, effectively relieving symptoms of PMS and other menstrual disorders without side effects. The next chapter shows how to use evening primrose oil as the foundation of a nutrition and lifestyle program that will minimize the symptom of PMS and other menstrual difficulties while maximizing your enjoyment of life.

RESOURCES

Further Reading

Lark, Susan, M.D. *Premenstrual Syndrome Self-Help Book*. (Berkeley, CA: Celestial Arts, 1993).

Ojeda, Linda. *Exclusively Female: A Nutrition Guide for Better Menstrual Health*, (San Bernardino, CA: Borgo Press, 1995).

Transitions
A monthly newsletter featuring self-help strategies for overcoming PMS. Published by
VizAbility Print Communications,
3119-43 Avenue
Edmonton, Alberta, Canada T6T 1C7
Tel. (780) 468-9633.
Subscriptions are $12.95 for 12 issues ($13.86 Canadian, $19.95 US for overseas subscriptions.)

Associations

National Women's Health Network
514 10th Street, N.W., Suite 400
Washington, DC 20004
(202) 347-1140
www.womenshealthnetwork.org

PMS Access
P.O. Box 9362
Madison, WI 53715
(800) 222-4767 or (608) 833-4767
www.womenshealth.com

Websites

Obgyn-net Women's Health Page
www.obgyn.net/women/women.htm

Women's Health Interactive
www.womens-health.com

4

The PMS Survival Guide

Now that we've explored the science behind
evening primrose oil and PMS, this chapter
explains how to use it in combination with other
supportive nutrients for maximum benefit. The
simple dietary and lifestyle strategies outlined in
this chapter offer additional help in dealing with
carbohydrate cravings, depression, fatigue, mood
swings, and temporary monthly weight gain.

A MODERN WOMAN'S AFFLICTION

PMS has become much more prevalent in the latter
half of the twentieth century, and not just because
it has been given a name and official recognition.
Studies done in 1934 found that 21 percent of
women suffered from PMS. Fifty years later, several large studies found that over half of the

women surveyed reported symptoms that qualified as PMS.

When you consider how the diet of the "typical" American woman has changed in the last fifty years, it's not hard to see why PMS has become a modern epidemic. In a misguided attempt at weight control, many women have eliminated much of the fat from their diet, in many cases replacing those fat calories with an equal number of empty sugar calories. But even more troubling is the fact that most of the fat consumed by American women today is either saturated fat from meat and dairy products or the unhealthful hydrogenated fats found in almost every processed food, quite literally from soup to nuts.

The end result is that today's typical diet is almost completely devoid of the essential fatty acids our bodies need to function properly. Few American women would consider themselves malnourished, but PMS is just one of the many health conditions that reflect this unsuspected nutritional deficiency.

USING EVENING PRIMROSE OIL FOR PMS

Evening primrose oil supplements are a safe and inexpensive way to supply the essential fatty acids you may be missing. They are readily available in health food stores, pharmacies, and vitamin retailers or from mail order sources listed in Chapter 9.

Recommended dosage: Begin with four capsules a day (500 milligrams each) and increase to eight per day if needed, taken half in the morning and half in the evening. Although it is not common, some people experience a slight nausea if they take the oil on an empty stomach. Taking the capsules with a meal usually eliminates the problem.

In some of the studies discussed in Chapter 3, the women took evening primrose oil only during the second half of their cycle, beginning several days before the symptoms were expected to start and stopping with the onset of menstruation. This approach is effective if you are concerned only with premenstrual symptoms. Given the wealth of other health benefits of evening primrose oil, however, many women continue to take supplements throughout the month, and there is no reason not to do so. In addition, because studies have shown that the benefits tend to increase with long-term supplementation, ongoing use may yield better results.

OTHER IMPORTANT NUTRIENTS

Several other vitamins and minerals are particularly helpful for women with PMS. Many of them are helper nutrients, or cofactors, needed to convert essential fatty acids to the beneficial prostaglandins. Taking them in addition to evening primrose oil ensures that your body has everything it needs to complete this multistep conversion process.

In addition, these nutrients perform many other important functions in the production of various hormones, the regulation of fluid levels, and the manufacture of brain chemicals that affect your mood.

VITAMIN B_6 (PYRIDOXINE)

Vitamin B_6 is a critical cofactor in the conversion of essential fatty acids into beneficial prostaglandins. In addition, it is helpful in clearing up premenstrual acne and acts as a natural diuretic, helping to relieve symptoms related to water retention.

B_6 plays a special role in the regulation and balance of female hormones. High levels of estrogen can have a dramatic impact on mood, causing anxiety, hostility, and irritability. Normally, the liver breaks down and deactivates excess estrogen in the bloodstream, but a deficiency of B_6 reduces the amount of estrogen that the liver can process.

Your body also relies on B_6 for the production of dopamine and serotonin, important mood-regulating chemicals. Numerous studies have shown significant improvement in PMS symptoms—especially mood-related complaints—with the use of supplemental B_6.

Because B_6 is easily destroyed during food processing, getting adequate amounts of this vitamin through diet can be difficult.

Recommended dosage: Supplementation with 50 to 100 mg B_6 a day is recommended as part of a nutritional approach to treating PMS.

MAGNESIUM

Along with B_6, magnesium is one of the most important nutrients available for the treatment of PMS. One of its many critical functions is to help to convert dietary B_6 to its active form. Even if you are taking in plenty of vitamin B_6, you won't get the full benefit if you are deficient in magnesium. Magnesium levels reach a low point during menstruation and diuretics used to treat water retention can further deplete these levels.

Women who have PMS tend to have very low magnesium levels and supplementation often brings dramatic relief from a wide range of symptoms. Magnesium can calm sugar cravings and regulate out-of-control appetites. By keeping blood sugar levels steady, it helps to head off the fatigue and headache that can be caused by the rapid rise and fall of blood sugar. Magnesium also reduces water retention and increases your ability to deal with psychological stress.

Recommended dosage: The recommended amount of magnesium is 500 to 1,000 mg daily. Magnesium is best absorbed when the stomach is relatively acidic and is best taken on an empty stomach. It is also a natural sleeping aid when taken right before bedtime.

VITAMIN B₃ (NIACIN)

In addition to playing an important role in fatty acid metabolism, vitamin B_3, also called niacin, is needed in order to make the sex hormones estrogen, progesterone, and testosterone. Niacin also helps your body convert carbohydrates into energy and can raise blood sugar levels. It can be very beneficial in the treatment of fatigue, irritability, depression, and intestinal problems such as diarrhea and constipation—all of which are common symptoms of PMS.

Recommended dosage: A safe dosage of niacin is 50 to 100 mg per day. For some people, niacin supplements can trigger warmth, redness, and itching of the face, neck, or other areas of the skin. This so-called niacin flush is a harmless and short-lived reaction and can be avoided by taking the niacinamide form of B_3.

VITAMIN C (ASCORBIC ACID)

Vitamin C fights inflammation by deactivating enzymes involved in the inflammatory process. It also is necessary for the production of beneficial, anti-inflammatory prostaglandins. Supplemental doses of vitamin C also can help regulate sugar cravings and related fatigue and headaches. Scientists who have studied cyclical breast pain and benign breast disease report that vitamin C taken in conjunction with evening primrose oil led to a significant reduction in symptoms.

Recommended dosage: Vitamin C is excreted out of the system relatively quickly. A daily intake of 2,000 to 6,000 mg should be taken in two or three divided doses. If you experience loose stools or diarrhea, simply reduce the dose to the maximum you can tolerate without adverse effects.

ZINC

This important mineral, critical in the conversion of fatty acids into prostaglandins, is frequently low in women with PMS. Alcohol consumption, stress, infection, diuretics, and/or birth control pills can all lead to a zinc deficiency. Zinc also can be depleted by high copper intake from foods, supplements, or water from copper pipes.

Recommended dosage: The recommended amount is 20 to 45 mg a day. Be sure to check to see how much zinc is included in any multivitamin you are taking and try not to exceed 50 mg total per day, in order to avoid imbalances of other minerals. Zinc is best absorbed on an empty stomach. If you are taking a separate zinc supplement, take it alone (first thing in the morning) for maximum absorption.

CALCIUM

Calcium is not involved directly with fatty acid metabolism; however, quite a bit of recent research connects calcium with a reduction of PMS symptoms. One of the largest studies, involving 500 women, showed that 1,200 mg calcium carbonate per day reduced such symptoms as mood swings, depression, water retention, and pain by half, after three months of treatment.

Recommended dosage: Very few women get the daily recommended allowance of calcium (800 to 1,200 mg a day), and chronic low calcium intake may be an underlying factor in PMS symptoms. Calcium intake is also very important for the maintenance of bone density and the prevention of osteoporosis in later years.

In addition to a daily calcium supplement, it is a good idea for women with PMS to avoid flavored soft drinks. The high phosphorus content of many carbonated beverages can seriously deplete calcium stores, by pulling calcium out of the bones and into circulation, where it is eliminated in the urine. Calcium-rich, naturally carbonated mineral water is a refreshing alternative.

DIET AND PMS

If you've ever doubted whether eating habits might contribute to PMS symptoms, consider these statistics. Women who suffer from PMS generally consume three *times more refined sugar* than other women do. Their diets are also 62 percent higher in refined carbohydrates (such as white bread, pasta, cereals, and crackers), 79 percent higher in dairy products, and significantly lower in iron, manganese, and zinc. (Zinc, as you'll recall, is one of the critical cofactors that your body needs to manufacture prostaglandins.)

Daily Supplements for PMS

Nutrient	Amount	Notes
Evening primrose oil	2,000–4,000 mg per day, divided into 2 doses	Start with the minimum amount and increase gradually if symptoms do not respond. Take with food.
B_3	50–100 mg per day	Choose niacinamide form if flushing is a problem. Take with food.
B_6	50–100 mg per day	Take with food.
C	2,000–6,000 mg per day, divided into 2–3 doses	If sugar cravings are particularly troublesome, the upper amount may be helpful.
Magnesium (citrate)	800–1,200 mg per day	Take between meals or at bedtime.
Zinc	20–45 mg per day	Take first thing in the morning.
Calcium	1,000–1,200 mg per day	Take between meals or at bedtime.

Diets that are high in white flour and refined sugar tend to be low in vitamins, minerals, and fiber. They are also notoriously low in essential fatty acids and high in hydrogenated fats and trans fatty acids. As discussed in Chapter 2, these artificial trans fats block the action of healthful fats and can prevent your body from making good rostaglandins.

But what do these statistics really mean? Does poor nutrition cause PMS, or does PMS lead to poor nutrition? Probably both. As you have already seen, low nutrient status is certainly a culprit in many PMS symptoms. But many women who eat an otherwise healthful diet find that their eating habits change radically during the premenstrual phase, driven by a ravenous appetite and/or uncontrollable cravings for sweets and starches.

PMS AND CARBOHYDRATE CRAVINGS

An intense craving for sweets and starches is a classic symptom of premenstrual syndrome. In one study, researchers found that women can consume up to 500 extra calories a day during the premenstrual phase.

While the body burns more calories during menstruation than at other times, due to a slightly increased metabolic rate, that may not be enough to compensate for the extra calories consumed—resulting in a net weight gain.

Another study found that, on average, women with PMS increase their intake of carbohydrates by a whopping 53 percent in the week before menstruation. Increased intake of carbohydrates, especially refined sugar, can make water retention more severe and increase mood swings and fatigue.

Many women also are plagued by guilt at their seeming inability to control their eating. But these patterns represent much more than just a monthly collapse of willpower. Sugar cravings are not merely a psychological appetite for women with PMS but rather a physical response to a chemical imbalance. The fact is that many women with PMS have an altered response to sugar called reactive hypoglycemia.

Women whose PMS symptoms include mood swings, depression, or irritability are the most likely to suffer from impaired sugar metabolism. At least part of this phenomenon may be the result of essential fatty acid deficiency. When the body is low in PGE1, it can become more sensitive to low blood sugar. Deficiencies of B vitamins and magnesium make the situation worse by lowering the amount of glucose (sugar) available to fuel the brain. The result is fatigue, headache, and a craving for sweets.

Although a sugar fix sometimes can bring temporary relief, giving in to the cravings can set in motion a never-ending cycle in which the more sugar you eat, the worse the cravings get. The supplement program outlined above helps to correct imbalances in the sugar metabolism pathway, breaking this cycle, and bringing relief for many women.

SEROTONIN AND PMS

Women who have increased appetite and cravings for sweets also may be feeling the effects of
low serotonin levels, which commonly accom-
pany PMS. A lack of serotonin in the brain can
cause feelings of depression, loss of concentration, apathy, and emotional volatility. Ingesting
large amounts of carbohydrates triggers the
brain's production of serotonin, with an almost
instant effect on mood and energy. While it may
be completely unconscious, women who eat
more sweets and starches during their premenstrual phase may simply be engaging in a form of
self-medication.

Unfortunately, the lift in serotonin levels after a
sweet snack is short-lived and the cravings are
back in short order, more intense than ever. Using
high-sugar foods to medicate low serotonin levels
can quickly lead to unwanted weight gain.

As we discussed in Chapter 3, drugs that raise
serotonin levels can be effective for the treatment
of PMS but can have unwelcome side effects.
There are, however, natural ways to stimulate serotonin production. (Before you begin treatment
with any nutritional supplement, consult your
physician.)

ST. JOHN'S WORT

St. John's wort is an herb that is now well known as a natural treatment for depression and anxiety. It is thought to work in a manner similar to the class of antidepressant drugs known as selective serotonin reuptake inhibitors (SSRIs). These drugs, which include Prozac, Zoloft, Paxil, and other "popular" medications, work by increasing the length of time that serotonin remains active in the brain.

Through its serotonin-boosting effect, St. John's wort can be very helpful in the treatment of PMS-related symptoms, especially mood disturbance and increased appetite. As an added benefit, the herb also helps reduce the levels of inflammatory prostaglandins in the uterus, which eases low back pain and menstrual cramps.

Recommended dosage: The potency of various St. John's wort products varies widely, so consult the labels for appropriate dosages. St. John's wort should not be taken in combination with prescription antidepressant medications, except under the direct supervision of your physician.

5-HYDROXY-TRYPTOPHAN

5-hydroxy-tryptophan, or 5-HTP, is an amino acid that directly stimulates the brain's production of serotonin. This well-researched nutrient has been successfully used in the treatment of many serotonin disorders, including depression, anxiety, eating disorders, and PMS.

Because of its potent effect on brain chemistry, 5-HTP should not be combined with other drugs, especially antidepressants, weight loss drugs, or alcohol. Taking 5-HTP on an empty stomach will enhance the serotonin-boosting effect.

Recommended dosage: Up to 200 mg a day of 5-HTP is safe for most people.

Both St. John's wort and 5-HTP are available over-the-counter from pharmacies, health food stores, and vitamin retailers—or see the end of this chapter for mail order sources. If you are taking other medications or being treated for a serious illness or chronic condition, please consult a health professional about the use of St. John's wort or 5-HTP.

A WORD ABOUT SAD

Seasonal affective disorder, or SAD, is a mood disorder that affects many people during the shorter, darker days of winter. Some people seem to be extremely sensitive to the decreased sunlight, which can affect hormone and neurotransmitter production. Symptoms of SAD, which include depression, lack of concentration, fatigue, and intense craving for carbohydrates, are familiar to PMS sufferers. Many women notice that their PMS symptoms are worse in the winter. In fact, there is some clinical evidence suggesting that women with PMS are more likely to suffer from SAD, and vice versa.

All of the nutritional strategies outlined in this chapter can be very helpful for people who suffer from SAD. Another effective treatment is the use of an ultra-bright light box—a tabletop appliance that emits extremely high-intensity light, simulating the effect of natural sunlight. Light boxes stimulate the pineal gland in the brain, restoring hormone and neurotransmitter levels to normal. They are also effective in relieving symptoms of PMS. For more information on SAD or light boxes, see the resource section at the end of this chapter.

EXERCISE

Add PMS prevention to the many benefits of regular exercise. Women who exercise regularly are less likely to suffer from PMS, and studies show that daily exercise significantly reduces symptoms in those who do. If you wait until PMS symptoms are in full swing, it may be difficult to motivate yourself to start exercising. But when you find yourself feeling grouchy, achy, or tired, try a brisk walk or some stretching exercises. Exercise is a terrific way to ease stress, reduce tension, and lift mood. It oxygenates the blood and muscles, increases absorption of some nutrients, helps to balance hormones, and stimulates the release of serotonin and other mood-enhancing chemicals. If you need still more motivation, exercise also lowers your risk of many common diseases, including heart disease, breast cancer, and diabetes.

Eight Diet Tips to PMS-Proof Your Life

1. *Limit consumption of refined sugar, which causes water and salt retention and increases urinary output of magnesium. Refined sugar also can exacerbate mood swings by causing a sharp rise and fall in blood sugar levels.*
2. *Limit salt to reduce water retention, especially during premenstrual days.*
3. *Avoid caffeinated soft drinks, coffee, tea, and chocolate. These all contain methylxanthine, a chemical that can provoke breast pain and tenderness.*
4. *Limit dairy to no more than two servings a day, especially if your premenstrual symptoms include anxiety and irritability. Too much dairy can interfere with magnesium absorption and reduce prostaglandin production.*
5. *Eat complex carbohydrates (whole grains, legumes, beans, and green leafy vegetables). In addition to being nutritious, complex carbohydrates help keep blood sugar levels steady and appetite in check.*
6. *Avoid foods containing hydrogenated or partially hydrogenated oils. These contain trans fats that*

can block the production of beneficial prosta-glandins.

7. *Increase intake of essential fatty acids by eating more cold-water fish, nuts, and seeds, to encourage the formation of beneficial PGE1 prosta-glandins.*

8. *Eat more fiber. Fiber regulates appetite, maintains regularity, and helps clear excess estrogen from the body.*

A FEW RECIPES (FOR ANY TIME OF THE MONTH)

Carbo-Craver's Breakfast Muffins

A high-carbohydrate, low-protein breakfast will help boost serotonin levels—and mood—throughout the day. These muffins emphasize complex carbohydrates, which give a more sustained energy boost and help keep cravings in check. Ground flaxseed contributes essential fatty acids along with extra fiber to regulate appetite and help maintain regularity. You can use preground flaxmeal or buy the seeds whole and grind them in a coffee grinder or blender. Ground flaxseed should be kept in the refrigerator and used promptly.

1½ cup whole-grain (or all-purpose) flour
½ cup oat bran
¼ cup ground flaxseed
½ teaspoon salt

  2 teaspoons baking powder
  ½ teaspoon cinnamon
  ⅓ cup raisins (optional)
  1 egg
  3 tablespoons molasses or honey
  ¾ cup prune juice, apple juice, or soy milk
  2 tablespoons canola or grapeseed oil

Mix dry ingredients and raisins, if desired, in a large bowl and set aside. Combine egg, molasses, juice, and oil and blend with a wire whisk or fork. Stir liquid mixture into dry ingredients and mix quickly in a few strokes. Bake in a greased muffin tin at 400° for 20 to 25 minutes. Makes 12 muffins.

Watershed Salad

This elegant and nutritious salad helps reduce water retention and bloating with vegetables that are naturally diuretic. Dandelion greens make a delightful salad addition, with a rich, slightly bitter flavor. You can harvest your own greens from wild-growing plants, but only if you are sure they have not been treated with chemical lawn fertilizer or weed killer. The smaller, younger leaves are more tender. Oranges are a good source of potassium and help to keep mineral levels balanced while excess fluid is shed.

  1 pound fresh asparagus
  2 fresh oranges

*½ pound fresh field salad or mixed
greens, including dandelion if available
Essential Balance™ Vinaigrette (see
below)*

Wash asparagus thoroughly and trim the tough
ends. Steam the stalks over boiling water for 5
minutes or until tender-crisp. (Do not overcook
the asparagus; it should retain its bright green
color.) Remove asparagus from heat and chill.
Peel and section oranges, slicing each section in
half and removing any seeds. To serve, arrange
chilled asparagus spears and orange sections
atop each serving of salad greens and drizzle
with Essential Balance™ Vinaigrette. Makes
approximately 4 servings.

Essential Balance™ Vinaigrette
This salad dressing uses an organic oil blend
made from flaxseed, sunflower, sesame,
pumpkin, and borage oils. In addition to a
delicious nutty flavor, this oil provides an
optimal balance of essential fatty acids,
including 28 mg gamma-linolenic acid per 1-
tablespoon serving. Look for this brand in
gourmet stores and health food shops. You
can also substitute another healthful oil such
as olive, canola, or grapeseed oil. Try to find
oils that are cold-pressed, minimally
processed, and packaged in light-proof containers.

> 2 ounces (¼ cup) Arrowhead Mills
> Essential Balance™ organic oil blend
> 4 ounces (½ cup) rice wine or cider
> vinegar
> 2 tablespoons chopped fresh parsley
> 1 teaspoon Dijon mustard
> 1 teaspoon sugar
> ¼ teaspoon celery seed
> salt and pepper to taste

Whisk or shake all ingredients together until blended and store in refrigerator for up to 2 weeks.

RESOURCES

Further Reading

ArgIsle, Bethany, and Brian Breiling, eds. *Light Years Ahead: The Illustrated Guide to Full Spectrum and Colored Light in Mindbody Healing* (Berkeley, CA: Celestial Arts Publishing, 1996).

Conkling, Winifred. *Secrets of 5-HTP.* (New York: St. Martin's Press, 1998).

Cass, Hyla, M.D. *St. John's Wort: Nature's Blues Buster.* (Garden City Park, NY: Avery Publishing Group, 1998)

Associations

Depression and Related Affective Disorders Association
Johns Hopkins Hospital
600 North Wolfe Street
Baltimore, MD 21287
(410) 955-4647
www.medijhu.edu./drada

National Organization for Seasonal Affective
Disorder
P.O. Box 40133
Washington, DC 20016

FULL-SPECTRUM AND HIGH-INTENSITY LIGHT INSTRUMENTS

Bio-Brite Inc.
4350 East-West Highway, #401W
Bethesda, MD 20814-4426
(800) 621-LITE
(301) 961-8557
www.biobrite.com

Light Energy Company
1056 NW 179th Place
Seattle, WA 98177
(800) LIGHT-CO
no website

The Sunbox Company
19217 Orbit Drive
Gaithersburg, MD 20879
(800) LITE-YOU
(301) 762-1786
www.sunboxco.com

Verilux, Inc.
9 Viaduct Rd
Stamford, CT 06907
(800) 786-6850
www.ergolight.com

HERBS AND NUTRITIONAL SUPPLEMENTS (MAIL ORDER)

L&H
32-33 47th Avenue
Long Island City, NY 11101
(800) 221-1152
(718) 361-1437
www.bvital.com

Swanson's Health Products
P.O. Box 2803
Fargo, ND 58101
(800) 437-4148
(800) 726-7691 (fax)
www.swansonvitamins.com

VNF Nutrition
240 Route 25A

East Setauket, NY 11733
(800) 681-7099
(516) 689-7638 fax
www.vnfnutrition.com

Vitamin Shoppe
4700 Westside Avenue
North Bergen, NJ 07047
(800) 223-1216
(800) 852-7153
www.vitaminshoppe.com

Vitamin Research Products, Inc.
3579 Highway 50 East
Carson City, NV 89701
(702) 884-1300
(800) 877-2447
www.vrp.com

5

Relief from Asthma, Allergies, and Eczema

RUNNY nose, sinus headache, burning eyes, sneezing, wheezing—anyone who suffers from them knows that allergies, while only rarely serious or life-threatening, can make your life absolutely miserable. If trees, flowers, or grasses set off your allergies, your suffering may be seasonal, peaking in the spring or fall. But if you are sensitive to house dust, molds, or pet dander, allergies can be a year-round misery.

Allergies often appear and disappear mysteriously throughout the course of one's life. Many people outgrow childhood allergies only to develop other allergies later in life. A move to a new geographical location or even to an older home can trigger new allergies, or you may suddenly develop an allergy to a cat that has lived in your home for years. Experts estimate that there are between 35 and 50 million allergy sufferers in the United States, and this is probably a conservative guess. Although the number of sufferers is vast, modern medicine has very little to offer in terms of a permanent cure for this perplexing condition. Unlike antihistamines and decongestants, which treat only the symptoms of allergy, evening primrose oil actually can reduce allergic sensitivity by gently rebalancing the body's biochemistry.

ARE YOU "ATOPIC"?

Atopy is simply a medical term meaning *allergy*. Hayfever, asthma, and eczema are all very different types of ailments, each with different triggers, symptoms, and treatments, but medical scientists refer to all of these as atopic conditions because they each stem from the same type of immune-system malfunction.

Atopy tends to run in families. If you suffer from hayfever, asthma, or eczema, the chances are much greater that your children will also be affected by allergies, although they may not be allergic to the same things or have the same type of allergy as you do. The hereditary aspect of atopy is thought to involve faulty metabolism of essential fatty acids.

Research has shown that people with allergies tend to have quite high levels of linoleic acid and abnormally low levels of its metabolites, GLA and DGLA. This means that, while the intake of linoleic acid is adequate, the conversion to GLA is blocked in some way. As you recall from Chapter

2, linoleic acid is largely inactive in the human body until it can be converted to GLA and then to prostaglandins that control immune response and inflammation, among other things. Allergic individuals appear to lack the enzyme delta-6-desaturase, which is required to convert linoleic acid to GLA. Today's rising rates of asthma and allergy may be due to the fact that, as a result of dietary and other factors, poor fatty acid metabolism has become extremely common, even in those without a hereditary problem.

Naturopathic and nutritionally minded physicians have long favored evening primrose oil as a natural remedy for allergy sufferers. The prostaglandins produced from GLA have a natural anti-inflammatory effect that helps to reduce the severity of allergy symptoms. Although you may not think of allergy as an inflammatory condition, inflammation of the sinus membranes, bronchial passages, skin, or even the lining of the intestines plays a major role in an allergy sufferer's misery. At its most basic level, however, allergy is a misfire of the immune system. By supporting proper immune system function, evening primrose oil works to decrease allergic sensitivity in general.

The immune system stands guard against invasion of the body by foreign entities and destroys damaged or infected cells before they can cause widespread damage. In order to do this, the immune system has complex mechanisms for distinguishing friend from foe, knowing which cells do belong in the body and which cells require a defensive response.

Your immune system produces many different types of white blood cells, each of which has a different method of identifying and eliminating foreign substances, or *antigens*. Some cells, called phagocytes, simply engulf and digest any substance that doesn't belong in the body. Other types of cells, called lymphocytes, create antibodies that deactivate antigens. Once the immune system has developed an antibody against a certain antigen, the body will always recognize that antigen instantly as a "known offender," and the appropriate antibody will be released to deactivate it.

ALLERGY: MUCH ADO ABOUT NOTHING

The body's immune system can malfunction in three ways. It can fail to recognize or respond to a foreign substance, allowing the invader—a cold virus, a foodborne bacteria, or even a cancer cell—to set up housekeeping and slowly weaken or destroy the host. This is called immune deficiency.

Sometimes the immune system gets confused and begins to mistake friendly cells for enemies, launching an attack on the body's own tissues or organs. Autoimmune diseases such as rheumatoid arthritis, multiple sclerosis, and type I diabetes are all examples of the damage that can result from this "friendly fire."

Finally, the immune system may overreact to foreign—but harmless—substances, such as dust or pollen. In an allergy attack, the immune system declares the presence of pollen or animal dander to be an emergency, producing antibodies that flood the body with irritating chemicals called *histamines*. These chemicals trigger inflammation and increased mucus production in an attempt to flush the invader from the system. Not only can the symptoms of the allergy attack make you miserable, but this constant misfiring both distracts and depletes the immune system, making it more likely that it will be unable to protect you from things that really *do* pose a danger.

PICK YOUR POISON

The most common atopic reactions are triggered by something we inhale, ingest, rub against, or otherwise come into contact with. It is not clear why the body overreacts to some substances but not others, nor do scientists know why some allergic (atopic) people develop asthma while others get eczema. We do know that people with one type of allergy are more prone to develop others as well.

Common Allergic Triggers

Inhaled	Ingested	Contact
Pollen, mold spores, animal dander, dust mite droppings, chemicals	Shellfish, peanuts, milk	Animal fur or saliva, grasses, cosmetics, latex, detergents

The most common allergic reactions, such as allergic rhinitis, asthma, and eczema, involve the eyes, nose, lungs, or skin. A systemic reaction such as anaphylactic shock is less common (but more dangerous).

Allergic rhinitis is characterized by a runny or stuffy nose, sneezing, itchy throat or eyes, dry or watery eyes, and swollen nasal passages. The most common triggers are seasonal pollens and grasses (hayfever), animals (most frequently cats, dogs, and horses), dust, dust mites, and mold spores. People with chronic allergic rhinitis often lose their sense of taste or smell, and can be plagued by halitosis (bad breath).

Asthma describes an allergic reaction that causes the bronchial tubes to swell and the tiny muscles that control the airways to spasm, causing wheezing and shortness of breath. Excess mucus production by the bronchial membranes also can hinder breathing. Asthma usually is triggered by the same sort of inhalants that cause allergic rhinitis, and many people with asthma suffer from both types of allergic reactions. Heavy exercise, sudden changes of temperature, and stress can all exacerbate asthma. This condition can be potentially life threatening and must be monitored carefully and controlled with medication, when appropriate.

Anaphylactic shock is an extreme allergic reaction that can cause respiratory or cardiac failure within minutes. Typically it is triggered by certain medicines, insect stings, or foods, such as peanuts or shellfish. Signs of anaphylactic shock include a rash or hives, difficulty in breathing, swelling of the tongue or in the throat, a rapid decrease of blood pressure (fainting), abdominal pain, and diarrhea. Anyone experiencing or in danger of anaphylactic shock requires immediate medical attention.

Eczema is an allergic reaction of the skin, causing severe itching and accompanied by red, rough patches. The rash typically appears on the face, the insides of the elbows, the backs of the knees, the neck, the wrists, and backs of the hands. It can be triggered by foods, inhalants, or contact with an irritating substance. Eczema is common in babies, especially those who are not breast-fed. Although it sometimes goes away within the first year of life, many people suffer from eczema throughout adulthood. The itching can be so intense that sedatives are necessary to control scratching, since excessive scratching can leave scars.

CONVENTIONAL TREATMENT OPTIONS

Most conventional allergists will suggest some combination of three treatment options: elimination or avoidance of the trigger substance, desensitization of the body's immune response, or drugs to mask or suppress the symptoms of allergic reaction.

AVOIDANCE OF THE TRIGGER SUBSTANCE

This is a fairly obvious solution, but unfortunately, sometimes it can be easier said than done. When a beloved member of the household, such as the pet dog or cat, is the problem, the solution may be confining either the pet or the sufferer to opposite ends of the house, or the heartbreaking decision of finding a new home for the pet.

Many sufferers invest in air filters and dehumidifiers to clean the air of dust, mold, dander, and other offending particles. Outfitting an entire home with air filters can be an expensive proposition, and, while it can make a significant difference, few people can completely eliminate their symptoms with these efforts because the particles have to be airborne to be pulled through the filtration systems. In fact, however, most of the most common allergy triggers are found in bedding, furniture, rugs, and curtains, and become airborne only when disturbed. When you sit on your sofa, pet your dog, climb into bed, or vacuum the rugs, for example, dust, mold spores, and dander are stirred up just long enough to come into contact with your mucous membranes and set off an allergy attack, before settling back into fabrics and out of reach of air filters.

Air filtration is more helpful for folks who suffer from seasonal allergies to grasses and pollens, which are designed by nature for air travel. But eventually everyone has to leave the house. Even a short walk or drive or a day spent in poorly filtered air of a school or office building can be a nightmare for those who suffer from hayfever. Although we don't tend to consider allergies to be a major medical problem, they are responsible for a significant number of missed work and school days during the height of the season.

To the extent that you can control your environmental exposure to allergens, avoidance requires knowing exactly what your allergy triggers are. The conventional method of testing for allergies, by skin-prick and scratch tests, is a tedious and inexact science. For one thing, allergies change as we get older and are exposed to different environmental triggers. Also, most allergic people have multiple and compound allergies. Cumulative and chronic exposure to allergens can cause your system to react to substances that might not have tested "positive" as one of your allergic triggers. (By the same token, identifying and avoiding exposure to your major allergy triggers often reduces or eliminates your sensitivity to other irritants.)

DESENSITIZATION THERAPY

If you do undergo testing to determine your allergic triggers, often the next step is some form of desensitization therapy. The idea is to train the body not to react to the source of the allergy (ragweed, cat dander, etc.) by gradually exposing the body to increasing amounts of that substance. This therapy usually requires going to a doctor's office for weekly injections. This technique can take months and even years, and may require ongoing follow-up to be successful. Even with long-term treatment, the success rate of this type of desensitization is disappointing. For some of the most common allergens, like dust mites, the chances of successfully eliminating an allergy—even after investing months and years—can be as low as 50 percent and may not be permanent. Desensitization is generally not helpful for atopic eczema.

In addition to this conventional method of allergy desensitization, alternative medicine disciplines such as homeopathy, acupressure, kinesiology, and environmental medicine offer other desensitization techniques. For many people, these holistic methods have proven quicker and more effective than traditional desensitization shots—both in identifying the triggers and eliminating sensitivities. In the Resources section of this chapter, you will find addresses to contact for more information on alternative approaches to allergy desensitization.

MEDICATION FOR TEMPORARY SYMPTOMATIC RELIEF

Drugs are by far the quickest and easiest solution, and doctors frequently rely on them to control the symptoms of allergies. For those who suffer from allergic rhinitis (nasal or sinus allergies), there are oral antihistamines and decongestants and nasal sprays that suppress inflammation and histamine release. For eczema patients, oral antihistamines and topical steroid creams are the standard therapy. To control wheezing and prevent attacks, those who suffer from asthma generally rely on some combination of steroids and bronchodilating drugs, administered orally or with inhalers.

In addition to the allergy medications that your doctor can prescribe, the typical drugstore or grocery now offers scores of over-the-counter allergy remedies. These include antihistamines, decongestants, low-dose steroid nasal sprays and inhalers, and topical steroid ointments. However, these drugs provide only temporary relief of the symptoms and offer nothing in the way of a permanent solution for allergies. And the side effects, which include dry eyes, headaches, and drowsiness, can be so unpleasant that many people resign themselves instead to sniffing and wheezing their way through the spring, fall, or even the entire year.

A MORE NATURAL SOLUTION FOR ALLERGIES

Instead of using drugs to suppress allergy symptoms or attempting to desensitize the body's allergic response, allergen by allergen, many naturopathic physicians prefer to use evening primrose oil and other nutrients that support the immune system and modulate the allergic response.

By promoting the production of PGE1 prostaglandins, evening primrose oil helps to alleviate allergic symptoms in two ways. First, it helps to decrease the inflammation that accompanies an allergic response. Second, it has an immune-modulating effect, specifically influencing the white blood cells that regulate the production of antibodies and histamines. In addition, essential fatty acids are vital to the health of the skin and mucous membranes and can make these tissues less vulnerable to irritation.

Because of their inherited inability to convert LA to GLA, atopic individuals are generally very low in the PGE1 prostaglandins that help to control allergic response. As you might expect, supplementing with evening primrose oil has been shown to raise the blood levels of GLA, accompanied by significant improvement in allergic symptoms.

Of course, many nonhereditary factors also block the production of prostaglandins. A deficiency of other nutrients needed to metabolize fatty acids, alcohol consumption, chronic disease, and aging are just a few of the common problems that can inhibit our ability to process linoleic acid into bioactive prostaglandins. Evening primrose oil is nature's solution, providing us with the more active form of GLA, which the body can then easily convert to prostaglandins. As prostaglandin production increases, allergic reactivity and inflammation subside—without drugs or side-effects.

USING EVENING PRIMROSE OIL FOR ASTHMA AND HAYFEVER

Substantial clinical and anecdotal evidence exists from physicians and patients who have found that evening primrose oil can be very helpful for all types of allergies, including asthma and allergic rhinitis (hayfever). Often, patients using evening primrose for other conditions, such as premenstrual syndrome, are delighted to find that their allergies or asthma also improve.

Recommended dosage: Physicians recommend 2,000 mg (four 500-mg capsules) per day for allergy sufferers.

In addition to essential fatty acids, several other nutrients have been shown to be helpful in controlling allergies.

OTHER IMPORTANT NUTRIENTS

VITAMIN A

Vitamin A is very important for general immune system support. Chronic allergies can deplete the immune system's reserves and leave the allergy sufferer vulnerable to infection. Vitamin A helps protect our vision, heal wounds, protect against infection, keep mucous membranes and skin healthy, and fight free radical production. Vitamin A deficiency is fairly common, largely due to inadequate consumption of fresh fruits and vegetables. Because vitamin A is one of the fat-soluble vitamins, a deficiency of fatty acids can also impair absorption of this vitamin.

Vitamin A is often formulated together with mixed natural carotenoids, which enhance its bioavailability and effectiveness. Carotenoids are natural precursors to vitamin A, found in deeply pigmented fruits and vegetables (carrots, canteloupe, sweet potatoes, leafy greens, etc.).

Recommended dosage: In addition to increasing your intake of foods rich in vitamin A, doctors recommend the addition of 10,000 International Units (IU) of vitamin A and up to 25,000 IU of mixed carotenoids through supplements.

B VITAMINS

B vitamins are necessary for the conversion of essential fatty acids to anti-inflammatory and immune-regulating prostaglandins. B_5 (pantothenic acid) helps reduce allergic symptoms directly through its anti-inflammatory effects. It also supports the adrenal glands, which can be weakened by chronic allergies. Folic acid, B_6, and B_{12} all support the antibody-producing arm of the immune system, helping to modulate allergic response. B vitamins are easily destroyed in food processing and deficiency is common.

Recommended dosage: 100 mg a day of a B complex vitamin.

VITAMIN C

Vitamin C is a natural antihistamine. It also stimulates the adrenal glands. Formulas that combine C with bioflavanoids are better absorbed. Bioflavanoids are natural plant chemicals found in citrus pulp and other fruit fibers. In addition to acting as cofactors that enhance absorption of vitamin C, they offer additional health benefits. *Quercetin*, for example, is a bioflavanoid that is frequently used to treat allergy.

Recommended dosage: Very high doses of C (up to 10,000 mg a day) can be helpful during acute attacks or at the height of allergy season. If these doses create intestinal discomfort (gas, bloating, and diarrhea), simply reduce the dose to a level that ensures bowel tolerance. You may be able to tolerate higher doses of C if you raise the dose gradually. The body excretes excess vitamin C quickly, so divide your daily dosage into several smaller amounts and take throughout the day.

ZINC

Zinc is needed to enable the liver to release stored vitamin A for use in the tissues. It is also anti-inflammatory and immune stimulating and aids in the metabolism of essential fatty acids. Zinc can be depleted by excess copper intake from foods, supplements, or even water from copper pipes. If possible, zinc should be taken on an empty stomach, without other minerals that may compete for absorption.

Recommended dosage: 20–45 mg a day is the recommended amount.

QUERCETIN

Quercetin is a naturally occurring chemical found in the rinds of citrus fruit, grape skins, onions, rhubarbs, and other plants. Closely related to vitamin C, quercetin is a very effective natural antihistamine and can be very helpful in reducing allergic sensitivity, including hayfever and asthma. It may take two to four weeks for quercetin to have an effect, so you may wish to begin taking it several weeks before you expect your symptoms will start.

Recommended dosage: 500–1,000 mg a day quercetin can be effective in reducing allergy symptoms.

Daily Supplements for Allergy Relief

Nutrient	Amount	Notes
Evening primrose oil	2,000–6,000 mg per day, divided into 2 doses	The higher amount is for eczema. Other allergies may require less.
A	10,000 IU per day, with up to 25,000 IU mixed carotenoids	Take with food.
B complex	100 mg per day	Take with food.
C	2,000–6,000 mg per day, divided into 2–3 doses	Increase amount to bowel tolerance.

Nutrient	Amount	Notes
Zinc	500 to 1,000 mg per day, divided into 2 doses	Can be taken on an ongoing basis, or beginning 2–4 weeks before your allergy season.
Quercetin	25–60 mg per day	Take first thing in the morning.

PROVEN RELIEF FOR ECZEMA

Numerous clinical trials have used evening primrose oil to treat atopic eczema, with mixed results. Some have shown remarkable benefit, others none at all. Analyzing the combined data from many different trials shows that, across many different study designs, evening primrose oil offers significant benefit for those suffering from eczema. While some of the criteria are somewhat subjective, such as an "overall impression" of improvement in the condition, others are fairly cut and dried, such as a reduction in the amount of steroid creams and other medications needed to control the symptoms.

Recommended dosage: It appears that the minimum effective dosage is 4,000 mg taken orally per day for adults. Greater improvement is seen with 6,000 mg per day, and the effect also increases with the length of therapy. Some of the trials that failed to note improvement may have used too small a dose or too short a treatment time.

A trial of sixty adult subjects with moderate to severe atopic eczema, conducted by Dr. Steven Wright at the University of Bristol, England, evaluated various dosages of evening primrose oil for their ability to relieve eczema. After twelve weeks, both the patients and their physicians noted a significant improvement in the symptoms, with reduced redness, scaling, and itch. Lower doses (4 500-mg capsules a day) led to only marginal improvement, but higher amounts (8 to 12 capsules a day) brought about much better results. Evening primrose oil was especially helpful in relieving the sometimes maddening itching that can make life miserable for eczema sufferers.

In 1990, based on the scientific evidence supporting its use, evening primrose oil was approved by the British Health Commission as a prescription medication for the treatment of eczema.

SOOTHING ECZEMA IN CHILDREN

Common in babies and young children, the intense itching and chafing of tender skin can make eczema particularly agonizing for both the young patient and for parents desperate to relieve the suffering. Although babies frequently outgrow the condition, this is small consolation to anxious parents, who are sometimes forced to use restraints to keep babies from scratching their skin raw.

Eczema is particularly common in children who have not been breast-fed or were breast-fed only for a few weeks or less. Breast-feeding is very important to the development of the immune system in babies, and an increased incidence of allergy, asthma, and eczema is only one of the consequences of insufficient breast-feeding of infants. In addition to important immune-building chemicals, breast milk is extraordinarily rich in GLA, which appears to provide significant protection against the development of allergic conditions. Unfortunately, most commercial baby formulas do not include these important fatty acids. (Japanese manufacturers have been the first to incorporate GLA and other fatty acids into infant formulas.)

Recommended dosage for children: Several trials have shown that evening primrose oil makes a safe and effective treatment for eczema in young children. Children as young as eight months old were given 500 to 1,000 milligrams evening primrose oil a day. (For purposes of comparison, a fully breast-fed infant takes in an amount of GLA equivalent to 2,000 mg evening primrose oil per day.) The children tended to show improvement even more quickly than adult subjects do, with dramatic improvements after only four weeks of therapy. Blood chemistry analysis showed that the supplements caused significant changes in the children's fatty acid profiles and prostaglandin activity.

For bottle-fed babies, capsules of evening primrose oil can be opened and mixed in with formula. Some researchers advocate using primrose oil topically in very young children, simply rubbing the contents of the capsules into the skin on the stomach or thighs, where it can be easily absorbed.

DELAYED FOOD ALLERGY—
A NOT-SO-DISTANT COUSIN

If you suffer from allergy, asthma, hayfever, or eczema, you are also more likely to be affected by something known as delayed food sensitivity. Unlike a classic food allergy (say, to peanuts or shellfish), which can trigger an immediate and obvious histamine reaction, delayed food sensitivities are much more subtle and often very difficult to diagnose. Symptoms, which can include gas, headaches, fatigue, or diarrhea, may appear hours or even days after eating a particular food. Although they are far more common than classic food allergies, many people don't realize that they suffer from delayed food sensitivities because they (or their doctors) never associate the symptoms with the cause. (Delayed food sensitivities are often misdiagnosed as irritable bowel syndrome [IBS] or spastic colon.) While food sensitivities represent a different kind of allergic reaction from hayfever or eczema, evening primrose oil can be very helpful in these cases as well.

An allergy develops when the immune system mistakenly produces antibodies to a harmless substance. There are several different types of antibodies, each of which has a different effect on the body. In the case of hayfever, asthma, eczema, and classic food allergy, the body produces a type of antibody known as immunoglobulin E, or IgE. These antibodies act on cells called mast cells, triggering the release of highly irritating chemicals called histamines whenever the offending substance is encountered. Typical allergy symptoms like runny nose, watering eyes, constricted bronchial passages, and itchy rashes are the body's reaction to a flood of histamine.

Delayed food sensitivities involve a different type of antibody called immunoglobulin G, or IgG. These antibodies can cause symptoms including gas, bloating, constipation, headaches, fatigue, water retention, or diarrhea. The problem is that it can take two or three days for the symptoms to develop, making it nearly impossible to connect the symptoms with the food that triggered them.

Until recently, identifying food sensitivities was a difficult and inexact process. Typical allergy tests are not helpful because they respond only to the presence of IgE antibodies in the blood. Newer, more sensitive tests have been developed to screen for the IgG antibodies responsible for delayed food reactions. (See the Resources section at the end of this chapter for more information on this type of test.) Once you have identified your trigger foods, symptoms usually can be improved or eliminated by completely avoiding that food for a period of time. Many times the food can be gradually reintroduced without triggering allergic reactions. Rotating foods, or avoiding eating the same foods day after day, can keep the immune system from redeveloping an allergic sensitivity.

A LEAKY WHAT?

Food sensitivities frequently are aggravated by something called leaky gut syndrome. Normally, the digestive tract is lined with slippery mucus-secreting cells that form an impenetrable barrier that keeps food and digestive juices sealed in the intestines. After the food has been broken down, nutrients are absorbed into the bloodstream through the lining of the small intestine, and all of the remaining material is escorted out of the body via the colon. The problem starts when tiny holes or perforations develop in the digestive tract lining, allowing small particles of undigested food to leak through the gut into the bloodstream. Even when the foods are perfectly healthful and nutritious foods, the immune system identifies the partially digested food particle as a foreign invader and mounts a defensive response.

If you suffer from food sensitivities, the constant release of IgG antibodies can cause inflammation of the lining of the intestinal tract, which can makes a leaky gut even leakier, and the problem spirals downward.

Evening primrose oil can be helpful in the treatment of both food sensitivities and leaky gut syndrome. As you'll recall from Chapter 2, essential fatty acids are critical to the maintenance of healthy cell membranes. When we are low in EFAs, our membranes tend to be leakier. The essential fatty acids in evening primrose oil help to repair the intestinal membranes, sealing the tiny perforations and restoring the integrity of the small intestine. By increasing PGE1 production, evening primrose oil also has an anti-inflammatory and immune-modulating effect, that helps to reduce the body's defensive reactions.

Recommended dosage: The recommended dosage is 2,000 to 4,000 mg (four to eight 500-mg capsules) evening primrose oil per day. Other nutrients that are helpful in the treatment of food sensitivities and leaky gut include vitamins B_5, B_{12}, C, glutamine, and zinc. These nutrients assist fatty acid metabolism, tissue repair, and support healthy immune response. In order to facilitate more complete digestion and absorption of nutrients, digestive enzymes are also recommended frequently.

RESOURCES

Additional Reading

Braly, James, M. D. *Dr. Braly's Food Allergy and Nutrition Revolution* (Los Angeles: Keats Publishing, 1992).

Null, Gary, Ph.D. *No More Allergies*, (New York: Villard, 1992).

Cutler, Ellen. *Winning the War Against Asthma and Allergies* (Delmar-Albany, NY: Delmar, 1997)

Randolph, Theron, M. D. and Ralph Moss, Ph.D. *An Alternative Approach to Allergies* (New York: Harper and Row, Publishers Inc., 1990).

Associations

American Academy of Environmental Medicine
7701 E. Kellogg, Suite 625
Wichita, KS 67207-1705
(316) 684-5500

American College of Allergy, Asthma, and Immunology
85 W. Algonquin Road, Suite 550
Arlington Heights, IL 60005
unlisted
www.allergy.mcg.edu

The Nambudripad Allergy Research Foundation
6732 Beach Blvd
Buena Park, CA 90621
unlisted
www.naet.com

National Center for Homeopathy
801 N. Fairfax St, #306
Alexandria, VA 22314
(703) 548-7790
www.homeopathic.org

Testing for Delayed Food Sensitivity

AMTL Laboratories
1 Oakwood Boulevard, Suite 130
Hollywood, FL 33020
(800) 881-2685 or (954) 923-2990
(954) 923-2707 fax
www.alcat.com

Immuno Labs, Inc.
1620 West Oakland Park Boulevard, Suite 300
Fort Lauderdale, FL 33311
(800) 684-2231
www.immunolabs.com

Herbs and Nutritional Supplements (Mail Order)

L&H
32–33 47th Avenue
Long Island City, NY 11101
(800) 221-1152
(718) 361-1437
www.bvital.com

Swanson's Health Products
P.O. Box 2803
Fargo, ND 58101
(800) 437-4148
(800) 726-7691 (fax)
www.swansonvitamins.com

VNF Nutrition
240 Route 25A
East Setauket, NY 11733

(800) 681-7099
(516) 689-7638 fax
www.vnfnutrition.com

Vitamin Shoppe
4700 Westside Avenue
North Bergen, NJ 07047
(800) 223-1216
(800) 852-7153
www.vitaminshoppe.com

Vitamin Research Products, Inc.
3579 Highway 50 East
Carson City, NV 89701
(702) 884-1300
(800) 877-2447
www.vrp.com

6

Healing and Protecting Your Heart

IT may surprise you to learn that you do not have to eliminate butter, eggs, and meat in order to have a healthy heart. Nor do you have to adhere to extremely low-fat diets. In fact, one of the secrets to heart health is getting enough of the right kinds of fats, primarily the essential fatty acids found in evening primrose oil and other healthful oils.

Few people in their twenties are really worried about heart disease. At that age, the threat of a heart attack seems about as remote as the next Ice Age. As you enter your thirties and forties, however, the reality of cardiovascular disease becomes somewhat more vivid. You may worry about parents or grandparents with high blood pressure or angina, or even lose a relative or family friend to a heart attack or stroke.

But it is usually not until we are in our fifties and sixties that the sobering truth of heart disease comes home to roost. Suddenly this once-remote and abstract threat becomes the thing most likely to end your life. Sadly, by the time most people are truly motivated to pay attention to their heart health, much of the damage—to arteries, blood vessels, and the heart muscle itself—has already been done.

The good news is that the cause—and cure—of cardiovascular disease is largely within your control. The right dietary choices actually can lower cholesterol and blood pressure and protect the blood vessels from damage that leads to heart attack and stroke.

This chapter dispels many of the popular myths surrounding diet and heart health. It also offers a scientifically based strategy to promote optimal hearth health with delicious foods you may have thought were off-limits forever, along with targeted nutritional support to keep your arteries free and clear. If you are on prescription medications for high blood pressure or cholesterol, please let your doctor know about any changes you make in your diet and supplement program so that he or she can monitor your need for continued medication. Chances are that after putting this program into action, you will be able to reduce or even eliminate some medications—but please do *not* discontinue any prescription medications without consulting your doctor first.

HEART DISEASE: GETTING TO KNOW THE ENEMY

You probably have heard the statistics many times. Cardiovascular disease is the number-one killer in this country, responsible for almost one in every two deaths in America. Heart surgeries (heart bypass and angioplasty) are among the most frequently performed operations, and cholesterol and blood pressure–lowering drugs among the most frequently prescribed medications. As a nation, our medical costs for cardiovascular disease top $56 billion every year. Yet the fatalities continue.

Why are Americans succumbing in such alarming numbers to heart attacks and strokes, even despite all these drastic measures? After all, our heart muscles are well designed to pump blood for 100 years or more without wearing out. The problem is that various factors (mostly diet and lifestyle) cause our arteries to become clogged and hardened with fatty deposits and plaque—a condition called atherosclerosis. The heart has to work harder and harder to force blood through these narrowed blood vessels, which raises the blood pressure. Certain factors can cause the blood to be sticky, or more prone to form clots that stick to the fatty plaques.

Finally, an artery can become so congested that the blood supply to the tissue it supplies is completely cut off. With no oxygen reaching the area, the tissue begins to suffocate and die. If it is the arteries to the brain that have been clogged, the result can be a stroke. When the hardening occurs in the arteries that lead to the heart, the outcome may be a heart attack or cardiac arrest. Heart attacks cause over half a million deaths a year in the United States.

Atherosclerosis is an insidious condition. Over years and decades, the damage to arterial walls can advance to a critical stage without a single symptom. Often, a heart attack—or even death—is the very first warning of heart disease. But what causes plaques to build up and clog the arteries in the first place? The answer may surprise you.

CHOLESTEROL'S BAD RAP

For several decades, cholesterol has been portrayed as the "bad guy" of cardiac health, presumably responsible for the buildup of plaque in the arteries. Cholesterol-lowering ("statin") drugs and low-cholesterol diets are routinely prescribed for those whose cholesterol readings are considered to be dangerously high (above 200).

This approach now appears to have been misguided on a number of fronts. First, the evidence linking high cholesterol with an increased risk of heart disease is mixed. About half of those with heart disease actually have low to moderate cholesterol levels. And many people with high cholesterol levels live long and healthy lives with no sign of heart disease. While there appears to be some relationship between cholesterol and heart health, it is clearly more complicated than we have assumed. As you'll see, the *balance* of different types of cholesterol is more important than the total levels. But in order to get a true picture of heart health, many other biochemical factors need to be taken into account, such as the levels of various compounds such as triglycerides, homocysteine, and lipoprotein(a) in your blood, your blood pressure as well as lifestyle and genetic factors.

Second, evidence shows that efforts to lower high cholesterol have almost no impact on the rate of death from cardiovascular disease. In fact, for those over fifty, higher cholesterol levels are associated with a *lower* risk of death from other diseases. In view of all this, many researchers have begun to question whether the cholesterol-lowering drugs that are so widely prescribed may cause more problems than they solve. Not only have these drugs been associated with an increased risk of certain cancers, but they also have been shown to cause a decline in cognitive ability and to deplete the body of coenzyme Q10, an important heart-protective nutrient. (This depletion may explain why many long-term studies show that a significant number of people develop or die of heart disease soon after beginning cholesterol-lowering medication.) The truth is that these drugs may be far more of a risk to your heart health than the cholesterol they are designed to combat.

Finally, low cholesterol can be just as dangerous

as readings that are too high. Cholesterol readings of 160 or lower are associated with an increased risk of lung cancer, liver cancer, alcoholism, depression, and suicide. Cholesterol is an important factor in brain function—in fact, the brain tissue itself is over two-thirds cholesterol! Abnormally low cholesterol may impair the brain's ability to regulate and manufacture neurotransmitters; this impaired ability may explain the increase of depression, alcoholism, and suicide associated with low cholesterol levels.

CHOLESTEROL: THE BAD NEWS

Recent research has revealed that cholesterol becomes harmful only when it is oxidized. Recall our discussion of oxidized fats and free radicals in Chapter 2. Cholesterol is a type of fat, like any fat, it is susceptible to oxidation. When fats oxidize, whether inside or outside the body, large numbers of free radical molecules are produced, and these unstable molecules can cause serious cellular damage to blood vessels and other tissues. This damage (and not the cholesterol itself) sets the stage for atherosclerosis to occur.

Cholesterol can be oxidized either inside the body or as a result of food processing. High heat and exposure to air accelerates the oxidation of cholesterol in foods. Many processed foods, for example, use powdered eggs or milk, products with a far longer shelf life than the fresh ingredients. But the high heat used in the dehydration process oxidizes the natural cholesterol found in these foods. This oxidized cholesterol is exactly the kind that you *don't* want to set loose in your bloodstream. Avoiding these types of processed foods and eating a lot of antioxidant nutrients (from fresh fruits and vegetables or from dietary supplements) helps to minimize oxidative damage to cholesterol inside your body.

THE GOOD NEWS ABOUT CHOLESTEROL

Far from being a villain, cholesterol is absolutely necessary for health, serving several important functions throughout the body. Most important, cholesterol provides the source material for the manufacture of steroid hormones such as testosterone, estrogen, and adrenal hormones. Cholesterol is also needed to make bile acids that are crucial to the proper digestion and absorption of other fats in our diet.

Cholesterol is found in many foods, including butter, cheese, cream, shrimp, and meats. And, of course, the richest dietary source of cholesterol is the notorious egg. Many people have been trained to believe that foods high in cholesterol are bad for the heart and that restricting dietary cholesterol will lower blood cholesterol levels. The truth is that avoiding dietary cholesterol has only a minimal effect on lowering blood cholesterol. Only a small percentage of the cholesterol we eat actually makes its way into the bloodstream. Most of it is broken down into smaller nutritional building blocks during digestion. These nutrients are then recombined into other molecules, and absorbed or excreted out of the body.

In fact, the vast majority of the cholesterol in your bloodstream is produced by your liver. The liver monitors the amount of cholesterol in the body and manufactures what is needed to maintain a certain level. Every day it synthesizes up to 2,000 milligrams of new cholesterol—equivalent to the amount found in about eight eggs. If you eat a lot of cholesterol, the liver will manufacture less, and by the same token, when you reduce your intake of dietary cholesterol, your liver steps up production to supply the difference.

THE STORY ON SATURATED FAT

Saturated fat, found mostly in meat and dairy products, also has been linked to heart disease, but as with cholesterol, the evidence is far from conclusive. Much of the initial research that linked saturated fats with heart disease actually was conducted using *hydrogenated* or trans fats. We now know that artificially hydrogenated fats are extremely unhealthy for the heart, but at the time of the initial studies, scientists didn't distinguish between natural and artificial forms of fats. Chapter 2 explained how trans fats block the body's assimilation of essential fatty acids, which have many heart-protective properties. It now appears that trans fats, not saturated fats, probably were responsible for the increased risk of heart disease observed in these early studies. By the time the distinction became clear, however, this dietary myth was firmly entrenched in the American consciousness.

It is true that a diet high in saturated fat tends to raise blood cholesterol, while essential fatty acids like evening primrose oil lower cholesterol levels. And this fact actually may be the key to the saturated fat and cholesterol enigma. People who are getting the majority of their fat calories from saturated fat or trans fats probably are not getting sufficient amounts of the heart-protective EFAs. A deficiency of essential fatty acids, not just the saturated fats themselves, may be what leads to high cholesterol. By the same token, a deficiency of EFAs—far more than saturated fat or high cholesterol levels—may be the true risk factor in heart disease.

This explains why the Inuit community, despite a diet that is extremely high in saturated fat and cholesterol, also enjoys one of the lowest rates of cardiovascular disease in the world. It also helps to explain why, despite the widespread use of cholesterol-lowering drugs and the promotion of low-fat, cholesterol-free diet foods, heart disease remains our nation's number-one killer. The essential difference appears to be that the traditional Inuit diet is also extremely rich in essential fatty acids.

Our goal in protecting heart health should be to

stop worrying so much about cholesterol and to start worrying about essential fatty acids. As you'll see, when you add EFAs like evening primrose oil to the diet, your cholesterol levels will tend to take care of themselves—no matter how much cholesterol you eat.

FAT IS HEART HEALTHY

Several very famous doctors have developed dietary programs reputed to cure and prevent heart disease. These diets are almost completely cholesterol free in addition to being extremely low fat, getting as little as 10 percent of their calories from fat. While these deprivation diets have shown some success in lowering cardiovascular risk factors such as high blood pressure and high cholesterol, followers of these types of regimens sometimes develop rather dramatic signs of essential fatty acid deficiency.

The truth is that it is not necessary to cut all fat and cholesterol from your diet to protect your heart. The success of the extremely low-fat diet probably lies more in the fact that these regimens effectively eliminate sources of unhealthful fat, such as saturated fats and the extremely damaging trans fats. But avoiding dangerous fats is only half the story. Adding healthful fats and essential fatty acids to your diet not only makes life a lot more fun, but it offers considerable benefits for heart health. In fact, researchers at the Harvard School of Public

Health recently concluded that "replacing saturated and trans unsaturated fats with unhydro-
genated, monounsaturated, and polyunsaturated
fats is more effective in preventing coronary heart
disease . . . than reducing overall fat intake."

Better Butter

*For decades we were led to believe that mar-
garine represented a heart-healthy improvement
over butter. But now scientists are telling us
that the hydrogenation process that turns liquid
canola or corn oil into solid margarine creates
dangerous trans fatty acids that can be more
dangerous than the saturated fats found in butter.*

*Here's a solution that wins on three scores. It
provides the incomparable flavor of butter but
with half the saturated fat and the added bonus
of healthful essential fatty acids. You'll also
appreciate the fact that it spreads easily directly
out of the fridge.*

*Unique among polyunsaturated oils, grape-
seed oil has been shown to improve cholesterol
ratios by raising HDL, or "good," cholesterol
in addition to lowering LDL levels. Grapeseed
is also naturally high in vitamin E, which protects it from oxidation. The best brand of
grapeseed oil is Salute Sante, which is processed
at low temperatures and shipped in UV-pro-
tected bottles. Ask for it at your local health
store or gourmet shop, or order directly from
the company at (888) 388-7117.*

2 sticks good-quality, lightly salted butter
1 cup grapeseed oil
¼ teaspoon salt

Blend all ingredients until smooth and spoon into a glass jar or plastic container, and keep refrigerated. Use in any recipe calling for butter or vegetable oil. Remember to limit total fat intake to around 35 percent of your total daily calories.

EVENING PRIMROSE OIL IS GOOD FOR YOUR HEART

Studies have shown that the essential fatty acids found in evening primrose oil benefit your cardiovascular health in several specific ways. As discussed in Chapter 2, the gamma-linolenic acid (GLA) found in evening primrose oil is converted to another fatty acid called DGLA in the body. Some studies have shown that low levels of DGLA in the blood and body fat is a stronger predictor of cardiovascular disease than the traditional risk factors (blood pressure, cholesterol, etc.). It also has been proven that evening primrose oil is the most effective way to raise DGLA levels.

To function at the cellular level, DGLA is converted further into the beneficial prostaglandin PGE1. Among its many functions, PGE1 regulates blood pressure, cholesterol, and blood clotting. Unlike cholesterol and blood-pressure–lowering drugs, however, evening primrose oil has no adverse side effects—in fact, it has a host of beneficial effects, such as reduced inflammation and enhanced immune function.

A NATURAL WAY TO LOWER CHOLESTEROL

Much research has been done on the ability of various polyunsaturated fatty acids to lower cholesterol. The essential fatty acids (linoleic acid and alpha-linolenic acid) both reduce cholesterol levels, but evening primrose oil is far more effective, and requires much smaller doses to achieve the same result. It appears that people with high cholesterol have difficulty converting linoleic acid (LA) to the more active gamma-linolenic acid, and then on down the metabolic pathway to the prostaglandins. Because evening primrose oil is a natural source of GLA, it overcomes this metabolic stumbling block and promotes an increase in cholesterol-lowering PGE1.

In one study, subjects who took 4 grams of evening primrose oil (eight 500-mg capsules) had an 18 percent decrease in total cholesterol. Subjects taking a much higher dose of linoleic acid only saw a 10 percent decrease in cholesterol.

Cholesterol is transported throughout the body as part of compound fat-protein molecules called lipoproteins. The two most familiar cholesterol types are called HDL (high-density lipoprotein) and LDL (low-density lipoprotein). LDL is often referred to as the "bad" cholesterol. This is the form of cholesterol that tends to build up on the walls of the artery, and can cause damage through oxidation. HDL, on the other hand, is often called the "good" cholesterol because it helps clear excess cholesterol out of the blood and transport it back to the liver, where it is metabolized and recycled. HDL also acts to protect LDL from oxidation. Recent research has established that the ratio of HDL to total cholesterol (HDL plus LDL) is a more accurate marker of heart health than the total cholesterol level.

Evening primrose oil lowers LDL cholesterol, while leaving HDL cholesterol levels intact (or only slightly reduced). The net effect is to increase the ratio of HDL cholesterol to total cholesterol levels.

Interestingly, when people with normal cholesterol levels take evening primrose oil, their cholesterol levels remain unaffected. This is because evening primrose oil, unlike cholesterol-lowering drugs, does not artificially lower cholesterol but supports the body's own cholesterol regulating mechanism. The result is perfectly calibrated cholesterol levels, neither too high nor dangerously low.

LOWERING BLOOD PRESSURE

High blood pressure is both a risk factor for and a result of cardiovascular disease. Blood pressure increases when the heart pumps a greater volume of blood through the arteries. High blood pressure puts a strain on the arteries and makes them more susceptible to tiny tears or abrasions in the arterial wall. These microscopic injuries can trigger the formation of plaques, as white blood cells, cholesterol, and platelets congregate and attempt to repair the damage. As arteries become stiff and narrow due to fatty plaque buildup, the heart has to work harder to pump blood through the constricted passage, which in turn elevates blood pressure even further.

One of the jobs of PGE1 is to regulate blood pressure, and evening primrose oil, by increasing the production of PGE1, has been shown to lower blood pressure in both human and animal studies. It can treat mild hypertension effectively and also protect the arteries from stress- or exercise-related surges in blood pressure. Again, while oils high in linoleic acid have some ability to lower blood pressure, evening primrose oil is far more effective. People with hypertension seem to be less efficient at converting LA to GLA. Evening primrose oil provides a supplemental source of GLA that helps promote optimal PGE1 levels and cardiovascular health.

DECREASES CLOTTING

Platelets are the cells that cause blood to clot at the site of a wound or injury to prevent excessive blood loss. Normally platelets go into action only if an injury occurs. If the platelets become too sticky, however, they can prevent the blood from flowing freely through the arteries and veins. In people with cardiovascular disease, the blood is frequently abnormally sticky and thick. Overactive platelets begin to stick to each other and to artery walls, and clots begin to form inside the blood vessels—especially anywhere that fatty deposits or plaques have begun to form.

Many people take a low dose of aspirin every day or two to prevent heart attacks. Aspirin works by decreasing platelet aggregation, making the platelets less sticky and prone to form clots. Aspirin is actually very effective at this task and is quite inexpensive. The downside is that daily doses of aspirin can cause damage to the stomach lining, even internal bleeding.

One of the benefits of evening primrose oil is that it is a natural inhibitor of platelet aggregation, keeping the blood slippery and flowing freely through your blood vessels and reducing your risk of a heart attack or stroke.

OTHER HEART-HEALTHY FATS

MONOUNSATURATED FATS

Monounsaturated fats, found in olive and canola oils, are heart healthy in many ways. First, they are more stable and resistant to oxidation than polyunsaturated oils, making them good choices as dietary and cooking oils. Monounsaturates have been shown to lower levels of LDL cholesterol and protect against the oxidation of cholesterol in the body. Those cultures that emphasize monounsaturated fats in their cuisine (notably Greece and Italy) enjoy much lower incidence of heart disease than other nations.

OMEGA-3 FATTY ACIDS

Many people take fish oil as a nutritional supplement for heart health. This became popular when researchers noticed that the Inuit have extremely low incidence of heart disease, although they eat a diet that is extremely high in fat and cholesterol. Other people who eat a lot of cold-water fish, such as Scandinavians, show similar immunity to heart problems. Further research revealed that two fatty acids found in fish oil, EPA and DHA, have many benefits for the heart.

You will recall from Chapter 2 that polyunsaturated fats are the source of two different kinds of essential fatty acids, the omega-6 family (which includes evening primrose oil) and the omega-3 family. Omega-3 fatty acids are derived from alpha-linolenic acid and are found in flaxseed, canola, walnuts, and soybeans in addition to cold-water fish like salmon, cod, tuna, mackerel, herring, and sardines.

Similar to the metabolic pathway that converts linoleic acid to GLA and then eventually into PGE1, omega-3 fatty acids are converted from alpha-linolenic acid, to EPA and DHA, and then on to another beneficial prostaglandin known as

PGE3. Both PGE1 and PGE3 have positive effects on cholesterol, blood pressure, and blood clotting.

The popular media has devoted quite a bit of attention to the omega-3 fatty acids found in fish and comparatively little to the omega-6 fatty acids found in evening primrose oil. As a result, the reputation of fish oil as a heart protector is well known, while the benefits of evening primrose oil are not. An important thing to keep in mind is that while the body can convert omega-6 oils into omega-3 fatty acids if necessary, it cannot perform the same trick in reverse.

A NOTE ABOUT FISH OIL

Many people find fish oil supplements difficult to digest—they are notorious for causing unpleasant "fishy" burping. Flaxseed oil is an alternative source of omega-3 fatty acids that doesn't cause this problem. Many people prefer to get their ration of heart-healthy EPA and DHA by enjoying salmon and other fish rich in omegas-3 on a regular basis (at least three times a week).

If you *do* choose to use a fish or flaxseed oil supplement, however, it is important to balance it with an omega-6 fatty acid such as evening primrose oil. Fish oil stimulates the production of beneficial PGE3 prostaglandins, but, taken in high amounts, it also can interfere with the manufacture of the more important PGE1 prostaglandins. By complementing fish oil with evening primrose oil, however, you will ensure optimal levels of both the beneficial prostaglandins.

Nine Diet Tips for a Healthy Heart

1. **Keep your intake of saturated fat (from meat and dairy products) to moderate levels**—no more than 7 to 10 percent of your daily caloric intake, or approximately 15 to 20 grams a day. Saturated fat tends to raise LDL cholesterol levels. But even more dangerous to the heart is the fact that when the body metabolizes these foods, it produces large amounts of an amino acid called homocysteine. High homocysteine levels increase the risk of cardiovascular disease by accelerating the oxidation of cholesterol.

2. **Avoid hydrogenated fats** like those in margarine, mayonnaise, shortening, and most processed snack foods. These artificially manipulated fats are extremely dangerous to the heart and to health in general. Trans fats raise LDL cholesterol levels and lower the level of HDL cholesterol. They also block the many beneficial actions of essential fatty acids by displacing them in the cells. Studies show that cooking with margarine almost doubles your risk of coronary artery disease.

3. **Avoid fried foods**, especially fast foods like french fries, fried chicken, and doughnuts. Restaurants use the same oil over and over again to fry foods. The repeated heating of the oil, coupled with the extended exposure to air, makes these oils, and the foods fried in them, a very potent source of dangerous free radicals that can damage your blood vessels.

4. **Avoid oxidized cholesterol** such as that found in processed foods containing powdered egg and milk products. Oxidized cholesterol can be extremely damaging to the walls of the blood vessels, causing blockages to form.

5. **Eat lots of fruits and veggies.** Fresh fruits and vegetables are rich in natural antioxidants that help protect the body from the oxidative damage caused by free radicals. Vitamin C, beta carotene, and selenium are all very potent antioxidants that are found in a wide variety of fruits and vegetables. Deep-green leafy vegetables are also a good source of B vitamins, which help to keep homocysteine levels in healthy ranges.

6. **Eat cold-water fish,** such as salmon, tuna, herring, mackerel, and sardines. They are all rich in omega-3 fatty acids, which have been shown to lower the risk of heart disease and stroke by reducing blood pressure, raising HDL cholesterol, and lowering the risk of dangerous blood clots.

7. **Use olive and canola as your main dietary oils.** These monounsaturated oils raise good cholesterol and lower bad cholesterol. They are also more stable than other cooking oils, such as corn and sunflower oil, and are less susceptible to oxidation. Cultures that eat diets high in monounsaturated fats have much lower rates of heart disease and other degenerative diseases. Aim for a total of no

more than 35 percent of your daily calories from fat.

8. **Enjoy eggs.** Because they are high in cholesterol, eggs have a reputation for being bad for the heart, but very little of the cholesterol they contain winds up in the bloodstream. A frequently overlooked fact is that eggs are also high in lecithin, a natural cholesterol-lowering nutrient that plays an important role in keeping cholesterol and other blood fats at normal healthy levels. Eggs are also an excellent source of good-quality protein.

9. **Eat more nuts.** Several large studies have found that people who eat more nuts have a reduced risk of cardiovascular disease. Nuts are high in monounsaturated fats and essential fatty acids.

NUTRITIONAL SUPPLEMENTS FOR A HEALTHY HEART

EVENING PRIMROSE OIL

Research clearly indicates that daily supplementation with evening primrose oil is beneficial in the treatment and prevention of high cholesterol, high blood pressure, and other risk factors for heart disease.

Recommended dosage: For general health maintenance and disease prevention, 1,500 milligrams a day (three 500-mg capsules) provides about 135 milligrams of GLA. When addressing existing cardiovascular problems, higher doses (up to 4,000 mg a day) can be therapeutic by stimulating increased PGE1 activity.

Other nutrients also work together to support heart health and function.

B VITAMINS

Homocysteine is a toxic amino acid that can build up in the bloodstream and accelerate the oxidation of LDL cholesterol within the arterial wall. High homocysteine levels have been linked to an increased risk of cardiovascular disease, heart attack, stroke, and Alzheimer's disease.

B vitamins, especially B_6, B_{12}, and folic acid, help your body to recycle harmful homocysteine into harmless methionine. B_6 is also an important cofactor in the process that converts the GLA in evening primrose oil to PGE1 prostaglandins and has been shown to have cholesterol-lowering effects.

B vitamins are naturally found in whole grains, beans, legumes, nuts (B_6); meats, especially liver, fish, eggs, and dairy (B_{12}); and leafy greens (folic acid). These water-soluble vitamins are sensitive to heat and light. Cooking and processing destroys many of the naturally occurring B vitamins in our food supply.

Recommended dosage: To lower homocysteine levels and support essential fatty acid metabolism, consider a mixed B vitamin complex or multivitamin, providing 50 mg B_6, 500 micrograms (mcg) B_{12}, and 400 mcg folic acid.

COENZYME Q10

Coenzyme Q10 is a vitaminlike substance found in every cell in the body. A potent antioxidant, coQ10 has a particular affinity for the heart and works to strengthen the heart muscle and improve cardiovascular function. CoQ10 helps protect LDL cholesterol from oxidation. It is also involved in the production of energy in the mitochondria of the cells and is reputed to increase general energy levels.

In the body, levels of coenzyme Q10 are regulated by the same metabolic pathway that governs the synthesis of cholesterol. Generally, the more cholesterol that is produced by the liver, the higher the levels of coQ10. One of the dangers of cholesterol-lowering drugs is that they also suppress the production of coQ10.

Recommended dosage: When selecting a coQ10 supplement, look for one packaged in an oil base, which will enhance the absorption of the nutrient. A general dosage recommendation for heart health is 100 mg a day.

MAGNESIUM

In addition to being necessary for the metabolism of essential fatty acids, this mineral has many important roles in supporting heart health. It helps to relax and dilate the arteries, allowing the blood to flow through more easily. Magnesium also prevents arrhythmia (or irregular heartbeat) and can help prevent spasms of the coronary artery that can cause angina or even a heart attack. Studies have found that heart attack victims have abnormally low levels of magnesium.

Natural sources of magnesium include nuts, seeds, legumes, soybeans and soy products, and whole grains. However, alcohol, sugar, and caffeine all deplete the body's reserves. The most readily absorbed forms of magnesium are magnesium citrate, magnesium glycinate, and magnesium aspartate.

Recommended dosage: For heart health, add 500 to 1,000 mg magnesium to your daily supplement program.

VITAMIN E

Of all the antioxidant nutrients, which also include vitamin C and beta carotene, vitamin E has particular heart-protective actions. Most vegetable oils contain small amounts of naturally occurring vitamin E, which acts as a preservative by protecting the fats from oxidation. Vitamin E has the same beneficial effect in the body, helping to prevent the oxidation of LDL cholesterol in the arteries.

Vitamin E also works to prevent the blood from clotting by inhibiting platelet aggregation, thereby reducing the risk of stroke and heart attack. Several studies have shown that vitamin E plays an important role in the prevention of heart disease, reducing the incidence of cardiovascular disease by well over half. According to the World Health Organization, low levels of vitamin E in the blood pose a greater risk for heart disease than high blood pressure or high cholesterol.

Recommended dosage: Recommended ranges for supplementation are 200 to 400 IU daily.

Daily Supplements for Heart Health

Nutrient	Amount	Notes
Evening primrose oil	2000–4000 mg per day, divided into 2 doses	Use the minimum amount for general prevention. Consider the higher amount if you have heart risk factors. Take with food.
B_{12}	500 mcg per day	Take with food.
B_6	50–100 mg per day	Take with food.
Folic acid	400–800 mcg	Take with food.
Coenzyme Q10	100 mg day	
Magnesium (citrate)	500–1,000 mg per day	Consume with a meal containing some fat to enhance absorption.
Vitamin E	400 to 800 IU per day	Take between meals or at bedtime

THREE LIFESTYLE FACTORS THAT MAKE ALL THE DIFFERENCE

Much of what we know about risk factors for heart disease was established decades ago by the famous Framingham study, in which Harvard researchers attempted to pinpoint which diet and lifestyle elements were correlated to the development of cardiovascular disease. Three so-called primary risk factors emerged from their analysis: high cholesterol, high blood pressure, and cigarette smoking. As we have seen, subsequent research has revealed that the connection between cholesterol and heart disease is less direct than previously thought, and, in many cases, high blood pressure is as much a result of heart disease as a cause.

QUIT SMOKING

The connection between smoking and heart disease is clear and uncontroversial. It's also the one risk factor that is within your own control. In the last twenty years, rates of heart disease and death from heart attack have leveled off, and even come down slightly, thanks mostly to the significant reduction in the number of adults who smoke. Smoking elevates cholesterol, raises blood pressure, decreases oxygen transport, and irritates the vascular tissue. Smoking creates extremely toxic free radical molecules that erode the lining of blood vessels and encourage atherosclerosis. These free radicals are also implicated in the development of lung and other cancers. If you smoke and are concerned about heart disease, the single most important thing you can do for your heart is to quit smoking.

EXERCISE

Like any muscle, the heart requires regular exercise to remain strong and healthy. Regular exercise increases the efficiency at which your heart pumps blood and oxygen through the system. It also serves to lower blood pressure and LDL cholesterol and to raise HDL cholesterol. Exercise also helps prevent obesity, which itself is a risk factor for cardiovascular disease.

Exercise can be as simple as walking a mile or two several times a week. In order to get the maximum benefit, however, you do need to push yourself to walk at a pace that significantly increases your heartbeat for at least twenty minutes. Less intense exercise is good for muscle tone, bone strength, and flexibility but will not necessarily benefit your heart.

LOWER STRESS

Another benefit of exercise is that it is an excellent stress reducer. Chronic stress plays a big role in the development of cardiovascular disease. Stress can raise blood pressure and also increase the release of stress hormones like cortisol, which lower the body's resistance to disease.

In addition to exercise, other stress management tools include meditation, massage, yoga and stretching, and creative hobbies such as cooking, gardening, writing, painting, and making or listening to music. Try to find a stress-relief valve in your life, and make it a point to unwind and relax often. It's not only good for your heart, it is an all-purpose recipe for a long and happy life!

RESOURCES

Further Reading

 Brecker, Harold and Arlene. *Forty Something Forever*, (New York: Health Savers Press, 1992).

 Charash, Bruce, M.D. *Heart Myths* (New York: Viking, 1992).

 Cranton, Elmer, M.D. *Bypassing Bypass: The New Technique of Chelation Therapy* (Troutdale, VA: Medex Publishing, 1992).

 Sinatra, Stephen, M.D. *Heartbreak and Heart Disease* (New Canaan, CT: Keats Publishing, 1996)

Associations

American College of Advancement in Medicine
P.O. Box 3427
Laguna Hills, CA 92654
(714) 583-7666
949 www.acam.org
Can refer you to a physician in your area who is certified in chelation, a natural, nonsurgical alternative to bypass surgery.

The American Heart Association
(800) 242-8721

The Institute of HeartMath
14700 W. Park Avenue
Boulder Creek, CA 95006
831 338-8700
www.heartmath.com
This research and education institute has developed innovative and scientifically proven tools for reducing stress and cardiovascular risk factors.

Nutritional Supplements

L&H
32–33 47th Avenue
Long Island City, NY 11101
(800) 221-1152
(718) 361-1437
www.bvital.com

Swanson's Health Products
P.O. Box 2803

Fargo, ND 58101
(800) 437-4148
(800) 726-7691 (fax)
www.swansonvitamins.com

Vitamin Shoppe
4700 Westside Avenue
North Bergen, NJ 07047
(800)223-1216
(800)852-7153
www.vitaminshoppe.com

Vitamin Research Products, Inc.
3579 Highway 50 East
Carson City, NV 89701
(702) 884-1300
(800) 877-2447
www.vrp.com

VNF Nutrition
240 Route 25A
East Setauket, NY 11733
(800)681-7099
(516)689-7638 fax
www.vnfnutrition.com

7

Hope for Chronic Diseases

EVENING primrose oil is perhaps best known as a natural remedy for premenstrual syndrome and atopic eczema and is becoming increasingly well known for its heart-protective properties. But there are many other troubling conditions that have been treated successfully using evening primrose oil, including schizophrenia, alcoholism, rheumatoid arthritis, multiple sclerosis, and other inflammatory and autoimmune disorders. Evening primrose oil has even been shown to have anticancer properties and is used in nutritional therapies for cancer patients.

As we have seen throughout this book, the widespread and largely unsuspected incidence of essential fatty acid deficiency is a common denominator in a surprising number of seemingly unrelated conditions. This chapter reviews the connection between EFAs and several of today's most prevalent and devastating illnesses and explains how evening primrose oil can make a significant difference in the course and outcome of these conditions.

It is perhaps worth repeating that the treatment of serious health conditions always requires the guidance of a qualified health professional. Although evening primrose oil often can reduce or even eliminate the need for prescription medications, especially pain relievers and anti-inflammatory drugs, *never* reduce or discontinue prescribed medication except on the advice of a doctor or other medical professional.

Quite a bit of research has been published on the medical applications of evening primrose oil as well as other nutritional and natural substances, but your doctor may not be aware of it. After all, no pharmaceutical sales representative is likely to have called your doctor's office to share the latest studies on evening primrose oil—while drug companies quickly bring to doctor's attention the slightest shred of scientific evidence in support of a pharmaceutical drug.

By sharing new information and your experiences with your health advisor, you may encourage him or her to become more aware of and involved in the great strides that are being made in nutritional medicine.

RHEUMATOID ARTHRITIS

Rheumatoid arthritis is similar to osteoarthritis (the more common wear-and-tear type of arthritis) only in that both diseases involve gradual destruction of the joint tissue. Unlike osteoarthritis, which affects almost everyone to some degree as they age, rheumatoid arthritis is an autoimmune disorder that can strike any time in life. Women are affected more often than men, and the disease can affect young children and teenagers.

WHAT CAUSES RHEUMATOID ARTHRITIS?

As discussed in Chapter 6, one of the ways in which the body protects itself is to produce antibodies against harmful invaders such as bacteria and viruses. For reasons that are not yet completely understood, in rheumatoid arthritis the immune system's antibody-producing machine gets confused and forms antibodies to the body's own cells—in this case, the synovial cells that cushion and lubricate the joints of the body. One theory suggests that infection with some sort of organism causes the body to create an antibody that not only locks onto and destroys that organism but mistakenly locks onto and destroys synovial cells as well.

Whatever the cause, the result is a relentless attack by the immune system on the body's own tissue, causing gradual, painful destruction of the delicate joint lining. Inflammation around the joints also results, which compounds the pain and leads to immobility. The most commonly affected joints are the wrists and fingers, resulting in the characteristically twisted and gnarled hands of a rheumatoid arthritis sufferer. Often the hips, knees, shoulders, and/or spine are also affected, which can leave the victim confined to a wheel-chair or even bedridden. In severe cases, the disease can attack other organs of the body, including the eyes, heart, lungs, and nerves.

Conventional medicine has no cure for this heartbreaking condition, which can cause mild to total disability and disfigurement. Strong steroid medications are used in an attempt to decrease painful inflammation, but steroid medications have serious side effects of their own, suppressing the immune system and leaving the patient more vulnerable to infectious agents or even cancer.

AN ALTERNATIVE TO STEROIDS

Evening primrose oil, on the other hand, is a non-toxic and harmless natural substance that appears to relieve the suffering of rheumatoid arthritis without the negative consequences of steroid med-ications. What we know about evening primrose oil and its ability to increase the production of PGE1 prostaglandins suggests that it can affect the course of rheumatoid arthritis in two important ways.

First, PGE1 produces a powerful anti-inflamma-tory effect that helps to reduce pain, tenderness, and swelling of the joints. (In this regard, it is quite helpful for those suffering from osteoarthritis as well.) People with rheumatoid arthritis tend to have elevated levels of inflammatory PGE2 prostaglandins, and supplying PGE1 to the body acts to decrease the release of PGE2.

Second, PGE1 modulates the immune system—specifically, it influences the production and activity of immune cells (called T-lymphocytes) that regulate the production of antibodies. In people with rheumatoid arthritis, these cells do not function properly. Evening primrose oil is helpful in the treatment of autoimmune diseases like rheumatoid arthritis because it helps to reduce excessive or inappropriate production of antibodies. Fewer antibodies means less destruction to the joint tissue.

You may wonder if decreasing the number of antibodies might weaken the body's defenses against disease. It's important to distinguish between a natural substance like evening primrose oil that brings the body's self-regulating systems back into balance and a steroid drug, which simply suppresses the entire immune system without discrimination.

Like any well-functioning government, the immune system has been equipped with many checks and balances. Some types of white blood cells step up the defenses against foreign cells, while others are responsible for calling a cease-fire when the threat has passed, to avoid damage to the body's own tissue. These cells communicate through various chemical signals. When this communication is disrupted, the immune system can get either overly aggressive, attacking the body's healthy tissue, or too passive, allowing invaders or cancer cells easy access.

Essential fatty acids, and the prostaglandins

they create, are a critical part of this communication. By providing the active precursor to PGE1, evening primrose oil helps the immune system restore and maintain a healthy equilibrium, with obvious benefit for those with rheumatoid arthritis and other autoimmune disorders (as well as those with underfunctioning immune systems, as discussed later in this chapter).

The widespread lack of healthy fatty acids in our modern diet, and our excessive intake of competing fatty acids such as trans fats, is quite clearly a factor in the increasing incidence of autoimmune disorders. It is also possible that those with rheumatoid arthritis may lack the enzyme necessary to convert linoleic acid in the diet to GLA, which effectively prevents their bodies from producing PGE1 in sufficient quantity to maintain a well-functioning immune system.

REVIEWING THE RESEARCH

Several double-blind, placebo-controlled studies have evaluated the effect of evening primrose oil on rheumatoid arthritis. In several studies, treatment with evening primrose oil markedly reduced morning stiffness and pain. One long-term study found that the improvement continued over the course of a year. In many of these studies, the patient relapsed when supplementation was stopped.

One of the most significant benefits seen in these trials was a reduction in the amount of nonsteroidal anti-inflammatory medication (NSAIDs) taken by the subjects. Sufferers of rheumatoid arthritis usually rely on heavy daily doses of NSAIDs like ibuprofen to manage pain and inflammation. These drugs work by inhibiting the production of the inflammatory PGE2 prostaglandins but do not increase the production of the beneficial PGE1 prostaglandins. The real problem with NSAIDs is the damage they do to the lining of the stomach and intestines. Many rheumatoid arthritis sufferers also develop ulcers due to constant use of these highly destructive compounds. Use of evening primrose oil offers a valuable way to decrease—or even totally eliminate—reliance on NSAIDs.

The various studies ranged in length from three to twelve months, and the most impressive benefits were seen in the longest treatment periods. If you are going to try evening primrose oil, don't get discouraged if you don't see profound results in only a few weeks. It may take several months to rebalance the system and turn things around. Also note that none of the trials to date reported any significant side effects, even in subjects taking very high doses of evening primrose oil over a substantial length of time.

Recommended dosage: 6 grams, or 12 500mg capsules a day.

OTHER HELPFUL NUTRIENTS FOR TREATING RHEUMATOID ARTHRITIS

Nearly all nutritional protocols for rheumatoid arthritis begin with evening primrose oil and other essential fatty acids like fish oil. Other nutrients known to be helpful include:

- Vitamin B$_5$: Helps promote the production of natural steroids by the adrenal glands.
- Vitamin E: Helps to combat free radical damage to the joint tissue and can help increase joint mobility.
- Zinc: Often low in rheumatoid arthritis patients. Zinc activates anti-inflammatory enzymes in the joints.
- Selenium: A powerful anti-oxidant. Selenium levels are frequently low in those with rheumatoid arthritis.
- Calcium (pantothenate): 2,000 mgs a day has been shown to reduce stiffness in rheumatoid arthritis patients.

RESOURCES

Associations

Arthritis Foundation
1314 Spring Street NW
Atlanta, GA 30309
(800) 283-7800

National Chronic Pain Outreach Association
7979 Old Georgetown Road, Suite 100
Bethesda, MD 20814
(301) 652-4948

The Rheumatoid Disease Foundation
5106 Old Harding Road
Franklin, TN 37064

MULTIPLE SCLEROSIS

Like rheumatoid arthritis, multiple sclerosis (MS) is a degenerative disease of somewhat mysterious origin that causes the immune system to wage war on the body's own tissue. "Sclerosis" refers to the hardening or scarring of tissue. In the case of multiple sclerosis, it is the myelin sheath that is destroyed rather than the synovial joint tissue. Myelin is a fatty substance that insulates the nerves and spinal cord. When this sheath is damaged, the nerve signals traveling through the body can "short out," causing widespread neurological malfunction. Symptoms of multiple sclerosis vary according to the location of nerve damage. Some people suffer only from mild "sensational" symptoms, such as tingling or numbness of the extremities. Others have motor impairment that affects their coordination, gait, or speech. Many others experience visual disturbances or loss of bladder or bowel function.

Multiple sclerosis is characterized by periodic "episodes," or attacks, with the first episode usually occurring between the ages of twenty and forty. Diagnosis is not an exact science. When presented with symptoms that are consistent with multiple sclerosis, a doctor will first rule out other possible causes, such as an acute viral infection or a tumor on the brain or spinal cord. When all other possibilities have been ruled out, a diagnosis of multiple sclerosis is given. Sometimes a computed tomography (CT) scan or magnetic resonance imaging (MRI) will show lesions or plaques on the brain and spinal cord, confirming the diagnosis, although these are not always present at the time of initial diagnosis.

The course of the disease varies widely. Some people experience only one or two episodes over a lifetime, from which they make a full recovery. Others have frequent episodes that may get increasingly worse and leave lasting impairment. The frequency and severity of the attacks generally predict whether the course of the disease over a lifetime will be relatively mild or severe. About 10 percent of those diagnosed with multiple sclerosis eventually will die from complications of the disease.

THE ESSENTIAL FAT CONNECTION

There are other similarities between rheumatoid arthritis and multiple sclerosis. In each case, researchers suspect that an unknown virus may play a role in the development of the disease. Both affect women in disproportionate numbers (although those men who do have multiple sclerosis tend to have more severe cases). Neither disease is curable, and both usually are treated with steroids to suppress the inappropriate immune response and slow the pace of degeneration. Interestingly, both rheumatoid arthritis and multiple sclerosis appear to be associated with the faulty metabolism of fats. Not surprisingly, both diseases have been treated successfully with evening primrose oil.

Since the 1970s, scientists have known that people with MS tend to have abnormally low levels of linoleic acid in their blood. During an active episode, this deficiency can become even more pronounced. Several studies found that supplementation with oils rich in linoleic acid, such as sunflower seed oil, was successful in reducing the number and severity of attacks in people with multiple sclerosis.

As you'll recall from Chapter 2, linoleic acid is biologically inactive in humans. In order to use this essential fatty acid, the body must first convert it to GLA, from which the body can manufacture valuable prostaglandins. Following the promising research on linoleic acid and multiple sclerosis, researchers hypothesized that evening primrose oil, as a natural source of the more active GLA, might be even more effective.

Animal studies have shown that evening primrose oil can stop the progression of autoimmune encephalomyelitis, the closest animal model to multiple sclerosis. And in several large surveys of multiple sclerosis sufferers, subjects reported that evening primrose oil improved or stabilized their condition. They reported fewer and less severe attacks and relief from symptoms, including increased mobility, reduced spasm or tremor, improved bladder function, and improved vision. Those who had taken evening primrose oil for the longest time reported the most improvement. For example, those taking supplements for four months to a year reported twice the improvement of those taking it for less than four months.

As we know, evening primrose oil promotes the body's production of PGE1 prostaglandins, and this is believed to benefit MS sufferers in several ways. First, PGE1 help to correct abnormal function of immune cells called T-lymphocytes. In autoimmune disorders such as multiple sclerosis and rheumatoid arthritis, certain T-lymphocytes, which are supposed to ensure that the body's immune system doesn't damage healthy tissue, seem to be defective. PGE1 helps correct this dysfunction and helps protect the myelin from overaggressive immune activity. PGE1 also enhances nerve signal transmission and the production of important brain chemicals called neurotransmitters.

Multiple sclerosis is also characterized by an abnormally high level of inflammatory prostaglandins. As you'll recall from Chapter 2, when essential fatty acids levels are low, the body's production of PGE1 suffers. Without sufficient amounts of PGE1, arachidonic acid is transformed into PGE2 at a much higher rate, causing a serious imbalance in favor of the inflammation-promoting prostaglandins. Although the body manufactures a small quantity of arachidonic acid on its own, most of the arachidonic acid in the body comes from meat and dairy products.

BALANCING PROSTAGLANDINS WITH DIET AND NUTRITION

Dr. Roy Swank is famous for developing a dietary approach that has had great success in relieving suffering and improving the expected outcome of people with multiple sclerosis. The Swank diet is extremely low in saturated, or animal, fats, based in part on the observation that multiple sclerosis appears to be more common in cultures that consume a lot of animal fat and less common in cultures where people consume a lot of polyunsaturated fats. It is thought that reducing the amount of arachidonic acid in the diet reduces the amount of inflammatory prostaglandins.

In addition to being low in animal products, and therefore low in arachidonic acid, Dr. Swank's diet is also very high in polyunsaturated fats, which promote the production of anti-inflammatory prostaglandins like PGE1. In truth, it is the level of PGE1 in the body that regulates the production of PGE2 rather than the level of arachidonic acid. Research has shown that arachidonic acid itself is harmless and leads to excessive PGE2 production *only in the absence of sufficient PGE1.* The key to the Swank diet for multiple sclerosis therefore may have more to do with its high essential fatty acid content than with the avoidance of meat and dairy products.

Supplementation with evening primrose oil is

another method of achieving the same goal and requires considerably less dietary restriction. Nutrition-oriented physicians regularly recommend evening primrose oil for the treatment and management of multiple sclerosis, in dosages ranging from 1,500 to 6,000 milligrams per day, or even higher.

Recommended dosage: The most common protocols specify 3,000 to 4,000 milligrams (that's six to eight 500-mg capsules per day). You can start with a smaller amount and increase the dosage if no improvement is noted. (Many studies have shown that people can consume up to 10,000 milligrams per day of evening primrose oil with no toxic effects, but obviously, if you can get good results on less, so much the better.) In evaluating your results, bear in mind that it may take from four to six months to see the full benefit of supplementation.

OTHER HELPFUL NUTRIENTS FOR HEALING MS

In addition, several other nutrients have been found to be beneficial, including:

- Coenzyme Q-10: This antioxidant nutrient improves tissue oxygenation and energy levels.
- Vitamin B_6: Important in the maintenance of nerves and nerve signal transmission.
- Vitamin B_{12}: Helps prevent nerve damage by protecting and maintaining the myelin sheath.

- Choline and inositol: Two additional vitamins in the B family that specifically protect the myelin sheath and support the
  function of the nervous system.
- Zinc: Those with multiple sclerosis are frequently deficient or absorb it poorly.
- Selenium: Frequently deficient or poorly
  absorbed by those with multiple sclerosis.

RESOURCES

Additional Reading

Swank, Roy L., M.D. *The Multiple Sclerosis Diet
Book* (New York: Doubleday, 1987).

Graham, Judy. *Multiple Sclerosis—A Self-Help
Guide to Its Management* (Rochester, VT: Healing
Arts Press, 1989).

Associations

Multiple Sclerosis Foundation
6350 North Andrews Ave
Fort Lauderdale, FL 33309
(800) 441-7055
www.msfacts.org

National Multiple Sclerosis Society
733 Third Avenue
New York, NY 10017
(800) 344-4867 or (212) 986-3240
www.nmss.org

Swank Multiple Sclerosis Clinic
13655 SW Jenkins Rd
Beaverton, OR 97005
(503) 520-1050
www.swank.org

SCHIZOPHRENIA

Although the causes of schizophrenia are not yet
known, modern medical science has made great
progress toward a better understanding of this
often-bewildering condition. Schizophrenia is
characterized by severely disordered thinking and
behavioral disturbances. Schizophrenics often suffer from hallucinations or delusions and may
become depressed to the point of catatonia or violent to the point of inflicting grave damage on
themselves or others. For centuries schizophrenics
were considered untreatable and confined to insti-
tutions for the insane. We now know that the
severe psychiatric disturbances seen in schizophrenics are related to biochemical imbalances of
the brain that often can be dramatically improved
with medication.

There are several theories about the origins of
schizophrenia, pointing to any one or a combination of triggering factors including viral infections,
head injury, traumatic experiences, nutritional
deficiencies, and metabolic disorders. It seems clear
that, whatever the trigger, the brains of schizophrenics produce too much of a neurotransmitter

called dopamine and that the resulting imbalance causes the personality and behavioral disturbances seen in these patients.

Dopamine-blocking drugs are often quite helpful in reducing the severity of the disorder, but the side effects of these heavy-duty tranquilizers can be devastating. Antischizophrenic drugs can cause symptoms that mimic Parkinson's disease, including tremors, shaking, and muscle rigidity. An even more debilitating effect of the drugs is a syndrome called tardive dyskinesia, which causes extreme involuntary movements of the head, neck, eyelids, jaws, and fingers. Unfortunately, many times the condition is irreversible even after the antipsychotic medications are discontinued.

Another promising avenue of research involves abnormalities in fatty acid metabolism that appear to play a role in schizophrenia. Schizophrenics have abnormally low levels of linoleic acid in their blood cells. In addition, they also tend to have low levels of some linoleic metabolites, including GLA and PGE1, and abnormally high levels of arachidonic acid and PGE2. From what we know about fatty acid metabolism, this seems to suggest that schizophrenics have some sort of biochemical abnormality in the way their bodies metabolize fats. Fat is essential for proper brain function; in fact, the brain is over 60 percent fat by dry weight and 20 percent essential fatty acids. Scientists have found striking differences in the types and amounts of fatty acids in the brains of schizophrenics and normal subjects.

These findings reinforce—and are reinforced by—the observation that schizophrenia seems to be related to excessive dopamine production. It is known that a decrease in PGE1 can be associated with an increase of dopamine release. Given its proven ability to correct faulty fatty acid metabolism and to stimulate PGE1 production in other conditions, evening primrose oil has been studied as a potential treatment for schizophrenia. Although it doesn't represent a cure, evening primrose oil has been shown to have significant benefit for schizophrenics, especially those for whom antipsychotic drugs have failed to control symptoms or who have suffered from severe side effects.

EVENING PRIMROSE OIL CAN HELP

Several clinical trials have evaluated the effectiveness of evening primrose alone and in combination with other nutrients and drug therapies. The most promising results were obtained using evening primrose oil in combination with penicillin (which also affects prostaglandin production) and in combination with nutrients that act as co-factors in the metabolism of essential fatty acids: vitamins C, B_3, B_6, and zinc.

The benefits were most pronounced in the reduction of so-called "negative symptoms" of schizophrenia, such as social withdrawal, depression, and unresponsiveness. Significantly, these types of symptoms typically do not improve with standard drug therapy. Evening primrose oil does not seem to be as effective against the so-called positive aspects, such as hallucinations or violent outbursts. These symptoms are not as closely correlated to abnormal fatty acid profiles and may be the result of other factors that contribute to this complex disease.

Another very promising finding was the ability of evening primrose oil to improve symptoms of tardive dyskinesia, one of the most dreadful side effects of the standard antischizophrenic drugs.

It appears increasingly likely that schizophrenia may not be the direct result of a single biological agent or dysfunction; more likely it has its roots in multiple interrelated factors. The most promising treatment avenues may be a combination of pharmaceutical, nutritional, and dietary approaches, fine-tuned to each patient's individual needs. A nutrition-oriented physician or mental health professional can help you design an integrated protocol. Among the other nutritional remedies that have been found to be helpful are:

OTHER HELPFUL NUTRIENTS FOR TREATING SCHIZOPHRENIA

- B complex vitamins: These cofactors are necessary for the proper metabolism of essential fatty acids into prostaglandins. B vitamins are also important in brain function and neurotransmitter production. Folic acid, one of the B vitamins, is found to be deficient in approximately one quarter of those hospitalized for psychiatric disorders.

- Magnesium: Also necessary for essential fatty acid metabolism and frequently deficient in schizophrenics. Magnesium also supports the action of B vitamins in maintaining brain function.
- Zinc: Often deficient in schizophrenics, zinc helps to balance out high levels of copper that are seen frequently in patients with this condition.

WHEN IT'S *NOT* SCHIZOPHRENIA

For a time, some scientists suspected that schizophrenia might be caused by an allergy to wheat. A wheat-free diet seemed to lead to dramatic improvement in some schizophrenic patients. It now appears more likely that these wheat-sensitive patients may have been misdiagnosed. An extreme sensitivity to gluten, known as celiac disease, can produce depression or even schizophrenic symptoms.

CELIAC DISEASE

Celiac disease is an inherited disorder characterized by an intolerance to gluten, a protein found in most grains, especially wheat, barley, oats, and rye. In addition to mood and behavioral symptoms, celiac disease causes damage to the mucous lining of the small intestine, impairing the body's ability to absorb nutrients from food. Because it is somewhat rare and difficult to diagnose, celiac disease often goes untreated. Over time, the condition can lead to serious malnutrition, even when a nutritious diet is consumed. Complete avoidance of gluten, although somewhat burdensome, usually results in a resolution of all symptoms.

DRUG REACTIONS

Several prescription drugs can cause schizophrenic behavior, including anabolic steroids sometimes used by body builders, cimetidine (the popular acid blocker Tagamet), ciprofloxacin (a wide-spectrum antibiotic), and others. And if that's not alarming enough, scores of other commonly prescribed drugs are known to cause confusion, delirium, disorientation, memory loss, paranoia, manic behavior, anxiety, and depression. Discontinuation of the drug usually, although not always, relieves the side effects.

EPILEPSY

Finally, a specific form of epilepsy called temporal lobe epilepsy often has been misdiagnosed as schizophrenia. In fact, research on the use of evening primrose oil in the treatment of schizophrenia led to an unintentional breakthrough in the diagnosis of temporal lobe epilepsy. Unlike true schizophrenics, who invariably improve or, at the least, show no change with the administration of evening primrose oil, those with temporal lobe epilepsy almost always get *worse* when taking evening primrose oil. It has been suggested that a trial course of evening primrose oil is an effective way to distinguish between those suffering from temporal lobe epilepsy and those who are schizophrenic.

Evening primrose oil has not been observed to cause adverse effects in other, more common types of epilepsy, and dosages of less than 6 grams (twelve 500-mg capsules) a day do not cause adverse effects even in those with temporal lobe epilepsy. Nonetheless, people with epilepsy should be cautious in using evening primrose oil.

Drugs That Can Cause Schizophreniclike Behavior

Amphetamine type drugs: Ritalin, Dexatrim, Dexedrine
Anabolic steroids: Halotestin, Android, Androderm, Testone
Cimetidine: Tagamet
Ciprofloxacin: Cipro
Ephedrine: Ephedron, Ephedrol
Phenmetrazine: Preludin
Phenylpropanolamine: Entex, Sinuvent, Triaminic Expectorant DH

RESOURCES

Further Reading
Pfeiffer, Carl. *Nutrition and Mental Illness* (Rochester, VT: Inner Traditions, 1988).

Associations

American Mental Health Foundation
2 E. 86th St
New York, NY 10028
(212) 737-9027

Celiac Sprue Association
P.O. Box 31700
Omaha, NE 86131-0700
(402) 558-0600
www.csaceliacs.org

Epilepsy Foundation of America
4351 Garden City Drive
Landover, MD 20785-2267
(800) 332-1000
www.epilepsyfoundation.org

National Institute of Mental Health
5600 Fishers Lane
Rockville, MD 20857
(800) 657-2642 or (301) 443-4513
www.nimh.nih.gov

National Mental Health Association
1021 Prince Street
Alexandria, VA 22314
(800) 969-6642
www.nmha.org

Well Mind Association
4649 Sunnyside North

Seattle, WA 98103
(206) 547-6167
www.speakeasy.org/~wma

CANCER

Evening primrose oil's potential as an anticancer agent seems to contradict directly some evidence linking an increased intake of omega-6 vegetable oils (those high in linoleic acid) with an increased risk of breast cancer in animal studies. More recent studies have determined that the connection between a high intake of polyunsaturated vegetable oils and an increased risk of breast cancer does not seem to hold true in humans.

In particular, numerous studies have shown the oil of the evening primrose to have significant potential in reducing tumors and preventing metastasis, not only of breast cancer but of many other types of cancer as well. Test tube experiments show that evening primrose oil inhibits the growth of every type of tumor cell tested, including carcinoma, adenocarcinoma, papilloma, melanoma, and sarcoma cells. When laboratory animals with cancer are treated with evening primrose oil, they consistently develop fewer and smaller tumors and have decreased metastasis and longer survival times. Evening primrose oil also has been studied in humans with cancer and has been shown to reduce the size of tumors. Much of the research has compared the anticancer effect of gamma-linolenic acid (GLA), found in evening primrose oil, to that of other essential fatty acid metabolites, such as eicosapentaenoic acid (EPA) and docosahexoaenoic acid (DHA), both found in fish oil. All showed varying degrees of tumor-fighting activity, but only GLA was both potent *and* selective. While EPA was active against tumor cells, it was not as selective as GLA; it also had an adverse effect on normal cells. Other fatty acids, such as linoleic acid and DHA, were simply not as effective.

Although there is still more research to be done, the use of evening primrose oil as both a cancer preventive and a treatment clearly shows promise. The exact mechanism by which evening primrose oil may fight cancer is not yet clearly understood. As in so many of the other conditions discussed in this book, cancer patients typically have very high levels of PGE2 prostaglandins and very low levels of PGE1. One of the functions of PGE1 is to stimulate the immune system; it could be that PGE1 deficiency is a factor in the immune system's failure to recognize and attack cancer cells in the body. Of course, as we know, evening primrose oil promotes the production of PGE1, which stimulates the immune system's defenses against cancer.

But there appears to be more to the story than the immune-enhancing activity of PGE1. Cancer cells have a much higher requirement for essential fatty acids than normal cells. The rapid division that characterizes malignant cells tends to use up certain enzymes needed to convert essential fatty acids to active metabolites, resulting in very lopsided fatty acid profiles. This in turn appears to make the cancer cells particularly resistant to oxidation, which makes them very difficult to destroy.

It is theorized that evening primrose oil, with its rich content of gamma-linolenic acid, somehow reverses this situation, effectively removing the cancer cell's bulletproof vest and causing tumor cell death.

Nutritional intervention in the form of dietary modification along with aggressive supplementation of vitamins, minerals, amino acids, herbs, food extracts, and other natural therapeutics has been shown to dramatically increase survival, enhance chances of attaining or sustaining remission, improve quality of life, and decrease the unpleasant side effects of traditional therapy. While we wait for further research on its potential as a primary therapy for cancer, evening primrose oil has an undisputed place as part of a nutritional protocol for the cancer patient. The topic of nutrition and cancer is far too large to allow a summary of other helpful nutrients here. The books listed in the Resources section offer more guidance.

RESOURCES

Further Reading
Diamond, W. John, M.D., and W. Lee Cowden, M.D. *An Alternative Medicine Definitive Guide to Cancer* (Tiburon, CA: Future Medicine Publishing, 1997)

Quillin, Patrick. R. D., C. N. S. *Beating Cancer with Nutrition*, (Nutrition Times Press, 1998).

Simone, Charles B., M.D. *Cancer and Nutrition* (Garden City Park, NJ: Avery Publishing, 1992)

Associations

American Cancer Society
1599 Clifton Road
Atlanta, GA 30329
(800) 227-2345
www.cancer.org

Cancer Information Service
National Cancer Institute
Building 31, Room 10A24
9000 Rockville Pike
Bethesda, MD 20892
(800) 4-CANCER
www.nci.nih.gov

Foundation for Advancement in Cancer Therapy
P.O. Box 1242
Old Chelsea Station
New York, NY 10113
(212) 741-2790
www.fact-ltd.org

National Breast Cancer Organization
212 West Van Buren Street
Chicago, IL 60607
www.y-me.org
(800) 221-2141

People Against Cancer
P.O. Box 10
Otho, IA 50569
(515) 972-4444
www.peopleagainstcancer.com

DIABETES

Diabetes used to be called sugar sickness. We now understand that this complex disease stems from a problem with the body's manufacture or use of a hormone called insulin, produced in the pancreas. In healthy people, food is digested and broken down into a form of sugar called glucose, which is absorbed into the bloodstream. A rise in blood sugar triggers the release of insulin from the pancreas. Insulin clears the glucose out of the bloodstream and into the individual cells, where it is converted to energy and used to carry out basic cellular functions. In diabetics, this process doesn't work correctly, and glucose is not cleared efficiently out of the bloodstream. The cells are deprived of the energy they need in order to function correctly. Moreover, chronically high levels of blood sugar can cause damage to organs and nerves throughout the body.

There are two types of diabetes, type I and type II. Type I usually is caused by an autoimmune disorder where the body's immune system attacks the insulin-producing cells of the pancreas. This type of diabetes usually strikes during childhood or young adulthood and almost always requires life-long insulin replacement therapy to compensate for a damaged pancreas. Type II diabetes (by far the more common form) is a condition usually diagnosed in middle age, in which the body becomes increasingly resistant to and unable to use the insulin produced by the pancreas. Type II diabetes often can be controlled by dietary manipulation to control blood sugar levels, but people sometimes need insulin to manage the disease.

Although the causes of the two kinds of diabetes are quite different, both can cause serious complications that can lead to kidney failure or blindness, or force the amputation of limbs. Chronic high blood sugar levels can damage the small blood vessels (capillaries) that carry blood to the peripheral nerves. Damage to the nerves in the retina can cause blindness. (Diabetic retinopathy is one of the leading causes of blindness in the Unites States.) Damage to the blood vessels supplying the kidneys can lead to kidney failure and death. Circulatory problems and nerve damage in the extremities, called diabetic neuropathy, can cause numbness, pain, or even the loss of a limb.

PREVENTING DIABETES-RELATED COMPLICATIONS WITH EVENING PRIMROSE OIL

While evening primrose oil can't correct the metabolic dysfunction that causes diabetes—namely the inability to convert sugar to energy in the cells—it has been shown to be very helpful in preventing or even reversing some of the dreaded complications. Both types of diabetes appear to impair the body's ability to convert linoleic acid into GLA, leading to chronically low levels of PGE1. New research suggests that the lack of PGE1 and a resulting imbalance in favor of the inflammatory PGE2 prostaglandins may be at the root of many of the most common complications seen in diabetes. As you may recall from Chapter 6, one of the actions of PGE1 is to dilate the blood vessels and increase blood flow and circulation. It is also critical to proper nerve signal transmission. In diabetes, supplementation with evening primrose oil, which increases PGE1 and suppresses PGE2, has been shown to improve circulation and to enhance nerve signal transmission.

A clinical trial involving more than 100 patients found that evening primrose oil improved the symptoms of diabetic neuropathy, including numbness and pain, and appeared to reverse some of the nerve damage that had already occurred and prevent further damage. Those who received a placebo instead of evening primrose oil showed significant deterioration of symptoms and nerve function over the same time period. After the first twelve months of the study, all of the subjects who had been receiving a placebo were switched, without their knowledge, to evening primrose oil supplements. Over the next twelve months, these patients also showed steady improvement.

Recommended dosage: 4 to 6 grams (eight to twelve 500-mg capsules) per day.

Evening primrose oil does not appear to affect or improve the diabetic's faulty blood sugar metabolism, but its ability to halt and reverse complications is a very significant step forward in the treatment of this increasingly common disease. A B complex vitamin, one that contains good amounts of B_{12}, also supports circulation and nerve function. Other nutrients, such as chromium picolinate, L-carnitine, zinc, and coenzyme Q-10, are helpful in improving glucose metabolism and blood sugar regulation.

RESOURCES

Further Reading

Whitaker, Julian M. M.D. *Reversing Diabetes*, (New York: Warner Books, 1987).

Philpott, W. H. M.D., and D. K. Kalita, Ph.D. *Victory over Diabetes* (New Canaan, CT: Keats Publishing, 1992).

Associations

International Diabetes Center
3800 Park Nicollet Boulevard
Minneapolis, MN 55416
(612) 927-3393
www.idcdiabetes.org

Juvenile Diabetes Foundation
120 Wall Street, 19th Floor

New York, NY 10005
(800) 533-2873 or (212) 785-9500
www.jdfcure.com

American Diabetes Association
1660 Duke Street
Alexandria, VA 22314
(800) 232-3472
(703) 549-1500
www.diabetes.org

National Diabetes Information Clearinghouse
2 Information Way
Bethesda, MD 20892
(301) 654-3327
www.niddk.nih.gov

ALCOHOLISM

Alcoholism is a steadily increasing problem in today's society, exacting a heavy toll on the health, livelihood, and life expectancy of the drinker. (Chronic alcohol abuse shortens life by an average of ten to fifteen years.) Alcoholism also places a burden on the families and communities of alcoholics, causing emotional pain, lost productivity, and often even posing a threat to public safety in the form of drunken drivers.

For a long time, an addiction to alcohol was largely considered to be a character flaw or a failure of basic willpower. But there is also evidence of a biochemical, possibly hereditary, component in this complex disease. No matter what the origin of the addictive behavior, stopping drinking can cause physical withdrawal symptoms and emotional anguish. Each case may be a unique combination of physiological, psychological, and social factors, which is why no single approach to overcoming this tenacious addiction has been universally successful.

Moderate to heavy consumption of alcohol—whether or not there is an addiction—is invariably deleterious to health. Alcohol affects every cell in the body, depressing the immune system, impairing brain and nerve function, and causing damage to the liver, pancreas, and digestive tract. Like most toxins, alcohol is broken down by the liver. Over time, chronic alcohol consumption can seriously damage the liver, inhibiting the production of digestive enzymes that the body needs to utilize proteins, fats, and fat-soluble vitamins. Malnutrition is common in alcoholics, not only because they may consume a large percentage of their daily calorie intake as nonnutritive alcohol but also because their bodies cannot effectively use whatever nutrients they are consuming.

Alcohol also blocks the conversion of linoleic acid to GLA, resulting in a deficiency of PGE1 prostaglandins. In fact, hangovers and the withdrawal symptoms experienced by heavy drinkers when they attempt to stop drinking may be related to extremely low levels of PGE1. A deficiency of these beneficial prostaglandins also increases the drinker's risk of lowered immune response, infections, cardiovascular problems, and brain and nerve deterioration.

Interestingly, small amounts of alcohol appear to have the opposite effect, actually increasing the release of PGE1. This could partially explain why very low to moderate alcohol consumption has been linked to increased longevity and lower rates of cardiovascular disease. The pleasant euphoria that accompanies moderate alcohol consumption also could be the result of increased PGE1, which stimulates the release of "feel-good" neurotransmitters.

Evening primrose oil has several potential applications in alcohol-related health problems. Alcoholism usually is characterized by an ever-increasing tolerance for alcohol. The long-term drinker often needs to drink larger quantities of alcohol in order to become intoxicated. In animal studies, evening primrose oil prevented the development of tolerance to increasing quantities of alcohol, which may help prevent addiction. It also helps to relieve depression and other withdrawal symptoms when heavy drinkers stop drinking, increasing the likelihood of long-term abstinence. In a study of 100 recovering alcoholics, those taking evening primrose oil showed improved liver function, improved brain function, and reduced withdrawal symptoms, including hallucinations, compared to those taking a placebo.

Recommended dosage: 2 to 4 grams (four to eight 500-mg capsules) per day.

For those who cannot or do not wish to stop consuming alcohol, evening primrose oil appears to have some ability to protect the liver from alcohol-related damage. It is also reputed to be an effective preventive and treatment for hangovers.

Finally, evening primrose oil may reduce the negative consequences of alcohol consumption during pregnancy. Fetal alcohol syndrome, caused by drinking during pregnancy, can cause a wide range of birth defects and abnormalities, including low birthweight, slow growth, mental retardation, and a higher infant mortality rate. It is theorized that alcohol, by blocking the conversion of linoleic acid to GLA, deprives the growing fetus of fatty acids and prostaglandins critical to its development. In animal studies, evening primrose oil prevented most of the alcohol-related abnormalities. This research must in no way be considered, however, to encourage or condone the consumption of alcohol during pregnancy.

RESOURCES

Associations
  Alcoholics Anonymous
  475 Riverside Drive, 11th Floor
  New York, NY 10115
  (212) 870-3400
  www.aa.org

National Clearinghouse for Alcohol and Drug Information
11426-28 Rockville Pike, Suite 200
Rockville, MD 20847
(800) 729-6686 or (301) 443-6500
www.health.org

National Council on Alcoholism
12 West 21st Street, 7th floor
New York, NY 10010
(800) 622-2255
www.ncadd.org

National Institute on Alcohol Abuse and Alcoholism
6000 Executive Boulevard, Suite 409
Rockville, MD 20892-7003
(301) 443-3885
www.niaaa.nih.gov

8

Looking and Feeling Your Best

MANY people are amazed to learn that fats can help them lose weight. After all, we've all been led to believe that in order to lose weight, we must eliminate as much fat from our diet as possible. And yet the fats in evening primrose oil have been discovered to be one of a dieter's best allies. (Not only that, but fat-free foods actually can make it *more* difficult to lose weight, for reasons you'll learn later in this chapter.)

Studies have shown that evening primrose oil supplements not only promote weight loss, but they can help you trim down even *without making any changes in your diet*. This benefit was discovered by accident during the course of a study on schizophrenics. Those patients in the study who were overweight by more than 10 percent of their ideal body weight (fifteen or so pounds) unexpectedly lost weight while taking evening primrose oil, even though they made no conscious changes in what they were eating. Subjects who were not overweight (or only slightly above their ideal weight) did not lose weight.

Recent research into the genetic and biochemical roots of obesity helps to explain how evening primrose helps your body burn up excess fat. Until fairly recently, the relationship between food and weight was regarded as a simple mathematical equation. As long as the number of calories consumed in the diet was equal to the number of calories expended by the body in its daily activity, weight should remain stable, or so the story went.

The number of calories in a particular food is a way of expressing how much stored energy that food provides. Once inside the body, food is digested and converted into energy as needed or stored as fat for future use. The old equation stated that weight gain was simply the result of consuming more calories than one expended and, conversely, that losing weight was simply a matter of decreasing caloric intake, increasing caloric output, or some combination of the two.

While valid to a certain extent, this formula leaves several unsolved mysteries. We all know people who can eat seemingly unlimited quantities of food without gaining an ounce. And there are also those who faithfully adhere to diets but don't lose weight. How can one person gain weight while eating exactly the same number of calories as another person who remains thin? Why do some people seem to have a much faster metabolism than others, regardless of dietary or exercise habits?

Bariatric science (the science of weight loss) has made important discoveries that make the old calorie/weight equation somewhat obsolete. While there is, of course, a connection between how much we eat and exercise and how much we weigh, we now know that the inability to lose weight is not always a failure of willpower. It is often the result of biochemical and even genetic influences that regulate our metabolism, or the rate at which our bodies burn and store fat.

IMPORTANT DISCOVERIES ABOUT THE FAT IN OUR BODIES

The body has two different types of fat cells, known as white and brown fat. White fat is so-called storage fat, the kind of fat that we associate with being overweight. When calorie intake exceeds calorie output, the excess energy is converted and stored in a layer under the skin until needed. All of us, even those who are very lean, have a thin layer of fat all over our bodies. In overweight people, excess fat tends to accumulate in thicker layers around the stomach, hips, thighs, and face. The goal of dieting is to encourage the body to use the stored white fat for energy, burning off the excess.

Brown fat, on the other hand, has a very different function. Instead of being a place to store excess calories for future use, brown fat is a specialized tissue that burns calories to create heat, a process called thermogenesis. This fat gets its characteristic dark color because brown fat cells have many mitochondria—tiny cellular furnaces that burn calories to create energy or heat. When functioning optimally, the thermogenic activity of brown fat can account for one quarter of the total calories burned off each day.

No matter how overweight we are, we don't accumulate additional brown fat. It is found in very specific places in the body: at the back of the neck, around the spinal column, and surrounding vital organs. In fact, brown fat itself is sometimes thought of as a kind of organ. Biologically, the brown fat appears to help us maintain body temperature and stable body weight. When it is functioning normally, brown fat will turn up the activity of fat-burning mitochondria in order to burn off excess calories that we may consume.

In trying to solve the mystery of why some people can eat more and gain less (and vice versa), researchers have discovered two very important differences between those who are naturally thin and those who have a congenital tendency toward obesity.

1. *Brown fat seems to be underactive in obese people.* For some reason, the mitochondria are not as active and do not burn off extra calories but allow them to be converted into storage fat. People with active brown fat cells burn up more of the calories they eat, so fewer are converted into white fat for storage.

2. *Obese people have lower levels of essential fatty acids in their tissues.* In fact, the association is inversely proportional: the lower the essential fatty acid levels, the higher the weight.

One of the functions of essential fatty acids is to maintain proper metabolism and thermogenesis. In overweight individuals, the prostaglandins produced from evening primrose oil appear to act directly on the brown fat, stimulating the mitochondria to burn more energy. This can transform a sluggish metabolism that seems to convert every calorie consumed directly into fat into a revved-up metabolism that burns off excess energy and reduces fat stores.

Evening primrose oil is especially helpful in stepping up the body's fat-burning capacity in those with a genetic predisposition to obesity. An abnormally slow metabolism causes these people to gain weight easily and makes it difficult for them to lose weight, even on low-calorie regimens.

Recommended dosage: The amount of evening primrose oil required to enhance thermogenesis is four to eight 500-mg capsules a day, or 2-4 grams. Because evening primrose primrose increases the basic rate at which the body burns calories, it can produce weight loss even without a change in eating habits. Combining evening primrose oil with a program of moderate caloric restriction and exercise can enhance the effect.

The New Science of Weight Loss: Supplements That Help

Evening primrose oil *promotes weight loss by turning up the thermogenic activity of the brown fat. The effect is particularly pronounced in those who are more than 10 percent above their ideal weight. The recommended dosage is 2 to 4 grams (four to eight 500-mg capsules) per day.*

Vitamin C *was shown to increase weight loss significantly in a placebo-controlled trial of forty-one obese people. Over a six-week period, subjects took 3,000 mg vitamin C (as ascorbic acid) a day but made no other dietary adjustments. Vitamin C also helps to reduce cravings for sugar and carbohydrates. The recommended dosage is 3,000 to 6,000 mg per day.*

L-carnitine *is an amino acid that is needed to transport fatty acids into the cells' mitochondria. It helps the body digest and use fats and helps break up fatty deposits. It aids weight loss and also increases exercise capacity and endurance. Red meat is the primary dietary source of l-carnitine, and deficiency is more common in vegetarians and those who consume limited amounts of red meat. Recommended dosage for l-carnitine is 500 mg daily.*

Chromium *helps to regulate blood sugar and prevent excess carbohydrates from being converted to storage fat. It also can help to control appetite and prevent fatigue following meals.*

Chromium levels tend to decrease with age, which may be a risk factor for adult-onset diabetes. Much of the natural chromium content of our food is lost in processing. The recommended dosage is 200 to 600 mcg a day.

Fiber not only regulates the appetite by making food more satisfying and filling, but it can help to block the absorption of calories in the intestines. Fresh fruits, vegetables, and whole grains are natural sources of fiber. A fiber supplement made with natural fiber from psyllium is another option. Total fiber intake should be at least 40 grams per day.

While evening primrose stimulates the brown fat to turn up the body's fat-burning furnace, very low-calorie diets tend to have exactly the opposite effect. Dieting actually can slow the metabolism— signaling the body to conserve energy and reduce the rate at which it burns calories—which is why most dieters eventually reach a plateau at which weight loss abruptly stops. Diets that are high in carbohydrates (including most low-fat diets) compound the problem by encouraging the body to store fat and further slowing the rate at which the body burns calories.

After years of fat phobia, in which the number of obese Americans has steadily increased, nutritionists are now beginning to understand the important role that dietary fats play in helping us achieve and maintain our ideal weight.

THE LOW-FAT LIE

For far too long, fats have gotten a bad rap where weight loss is concerned. The diet industry has convinced most Americans that they must elimi- nate fat from the diet in order to lose weight. There are even those that would have you believe that, as long as you don't eat any fat, you can eat as much as want without gaining weight.

Sometimes we imagine that the fat in our foods is deposited directly into our body's fat stores, on the hips, thighs, or wherever your body tends to store fat. But, of course, it's a little more compli- cated than that. The fats, proteins, and carbohy- drates we eat are all broken down into nutrients for absorption. Fats are broken down into individ- ual fatty acid molecules, proteins into amino acid building blocks, and carbohydrates into glucose. The body then recombines these building blocks into the proteins and fatty acids needed for tissue repair and maintenance and other functions. The cells use the glucose for energy. If the body ends up with more glucose than it needs to fuel its activi- ties, it stores the excess energy as fat until needed. So, as you can see, the pat of butter on your potato is no more likely to end up on your hips than the carbohydrates in the potato itself.

THE SNACKWELL SYNDROME

About ten years ago, this country began a low-fat feeding frenzy sometimes referred to as the Snackwell syndrome, named for the wildly successful line of low-fat cookies and cakes that launched the reduced-fat food craze. Today, despite the availability of low-fat and fat-free versions of virtually every food under the sun, Americans are heavier than ever.

What many dieters fail to realize is that popular reduced-fat products such as cookies, candy bars, peanut butters, and ice cream, are just as high or higher in calories than the original product. The fat calories have been replaced by an equal number of empty sugar calories, lulling many into a false sense of security. Research has shown that people who think they are eating low-fat foods overcompensate, eating more calories than they would if they thought the food was of normal fat content. But it isn't just a psychological trap. Even when people don't know whether the foods are regular or low-fat versions, those eating low-fat foods tend to consume more total calories. It appears that, calorie for calorie, low-fat food is simply less satisfying.

Part of the reason for fat's bad reputation is that it is relatively calorie dense. Gram for gram, fats provide more than twice the calories of proteins and carbohydrates. While carbohydrates and proteins have only 4 calories per gram, fats have 9 calories per gram. The low-fat advocates fail to take into consideration that, while fats are more calorie dense, they are also more satisfying, so we tend to eat less of them. A few fat calories can go a long way toward making our food more delicious and satisfying. It's no great feat to polish off 100 grams of carbohydrates (approximately two and a half cups of pasta). But few of us would sit down and eat 100 grams of fat (an entire stick of butter) at one sitting.

Carbohydrates simply don't satisfy the body's appetite the same way fats and proteins do. Although huge plates of pasta or large quantities of bread or potatoes take up a lot of space in the stomach, making you feel temporarily full, the body digests carbohydrates quickly, leaving you hungry after only a short time. Fats and proteins, because of their more complex molecular structure, take longer to digest, leaving you feeling satisfied for longer.

The fact is that fats are very important—especially for dieters—because they increase the satiety factor of foods. Because they are digested more slowly than carbohydrates, you go longer before feeling hungry again. But there are many other important ways that healthy fats can fuel weight loss.

FATS ACTUALLY CAN SPEED WEIGHT LOSS

You may be surprised to learn that, as long as your
total calorie intake remains low, eating more fat
doesn't hinder your ability to lose weight—in fact,
it may help. One weight-loss experiment conducted in Geneva, Switzerland, divided female
dieters into two groups, each of whom ate the
same number of calories each day (1,200). In one
group, the percentage of fat was kept to a low 26
percent, while the other group ate 45 percent of
their calories from fat. After three months, both
groups had lost the same amount of weight. In
fact, the group eating the high-fat diet actually lost
slightly more body fat than the low-fat eaters. (A
1,200-calorie diet is an extremely low-calorie diet
and is not recommended for long-term weight-loss
efforts, but, nonetheless, the results of this study
were quite interesting.)

One explanation for this surprising finding is
that an extremely low-fat, high-carbohydrate diet
appears to slow down your metabolism, decreasing the rate at which your body burns calories.
High-carbohydrate diets also can encourage your
body to make and store fat!

Many carbohydrate foods, particularly those
made with refined white flour and any type of
sweetener, are considered to be high-glycemic
foods. This means that they create a rapid rise in
blood sugar, which causes the pancreas to secrete

large amounts of insulin into the bloodstream. The insulin works overtime to clear the sugar from the bloodstream, which can leave you feeling weak, fatigued, jittery . . . and *hungry*. Insulin also instructs the body to store the excess carbohydrates as fat rather than burn them for energy.

Over time, this sugar/insulin roller coaster, besides promoting weight and fat gain, can have disastrous health consequences. In a condition known as Syndrome X, the body can become increasingly resistant to insulin, requiring more and more to restore normal blood sugar. Syndrome X is the first step toward the development of Type II diabetes and is a risk factor for cardiovascular disease as well.

One way to slow down the release of sugar from high-glycemic foods is to combine them with foods containing protein, fat, and fiber. These foods are digested more slowly and help to keep blood sugar levels more balanced. A balanced diet, including adequate protein and healthy fats in addition to carbohydrates, promotes the body's fat-burning mechanism instead of its fat-storing tendencies. Fat and protein also make foods more filling and satisfying, heading off hunger pains that can sabotage even the most determined dieter.

Good Carbs versus Bad Carbs

Perhaps the greatest pitfall of low-fat, high-carbohydrate diets is that they don't always distinguish between good carbohydrates and harmful ones. Just as there are both healthful and unhealthful types of fat, all carbohydrates are not equally nutritious. Some carbohydrates, such as fruits, vegetables, legumes, and beans, offer high-quality nutrition, including plenty of naturally occurring vitamins, minerals, and fiber, and are excellent choices for dieters. Other carbohydrates, especially the highly refined flours and sugars found in most processed low-fat treats, are essentially empty calories that do nothing but wreak havoc on your blood sugar and encourage fat storage.

LOW FAT IS UNHEALTHY

Not only do low-fat foods not make us thinner, they deprive us of all of the important health benefits of essential fatty acids. Over the long term, low-fat dieting can lead to thinning hair, dandruff, blemishes, dull complexion, and nails that refuse to grow. In addition, inadequate consumption of essential fatty acids can exacerbate ailments like arthritis and premenstrual syndrome. Most of these symptoms can be reversed rapidly by adding essential fatty acids, in the form of evening primrose oil, to the diet.

Some Problems with Low-Fat Diets

1. High-carbohydrate diets can be high in sugar, low in nutrition.
2. Too many refined carbohydrates can promote

insulin resistance, a risk factor for diabetes and heart disease.

3. Low-fat diets frequently are deficient in essential fatty acids.
4. High-carbohydrate diets tend to increase the appetite.
5. Low-fat diets slow the metabolism.
6. High-carbohydrate meals can cause a rapid rise and fall in blood sugar, resulting in fatigue and/or headaches.
7. Excessive carbohydrate intake encourages fat production and storage.
8. Carbohydrates promote water retention and water weight gain.

HEALTHFUL FATS FOR HEALTHY WEIGHT LOSS

With all the low-fat hype, you might be concerned that adding some fat to your diet will sabotage your efforts. In fact, you may find that eating more healthful fats make it easier to reach your goals. You're likely to be less hungry and feel less deprived. The right kinds of fat also will keep your fat-burning engines revved and help to prevent the dreaded weight-loss plateau. Finally, you'll have more energy and overall enhanced health. (If you are trying to reduce, it's important to watch your total calorie intake. You don't want to overindulge in fats any more than you want to overindulge in general.)

If you have tried to lose weight on low-fat diets and found that they were impossible to stick to

or just didn't work, you might be pleasantly surprised by your results on a more balanced regimen.
Many nutritionists are now recommending a diet
that consists of around 50 percent carbohydrates
(emphasizing vegetables, fruits, beans, legumes,
and whole grains and minimizing highly processed
flour and sugar-based foods), 15 to 20 percent protein, and 30 percent fat (emphasizing the healthful
unsaturated fats and minimizing dangerous trans
fatty acids).

The following sample menus using this balance
show how delicious and satisfying even a low-
calorie diet can be. Each sample day provides
approximately 1,600 calories (200 g carbohydrates, 80 g protein and 53 g healthy fats), which
would allow a 140-pound woman to lose about
one to two pounds a week.

Day One
    1 whole-grain bagel with 1 tablespoon cream
      cheese
    Roll-up or wrap sandwich, made with ½ cup
      prepared hummus, shredded carrots, and let-
      tuce in a whole-wheat pita or tortilla
    1 peach, plum, or fruit in season
    Stir-fry chicken and vegetables with peanuts
      (recipe follows)
    ½ cup rice
    2 fortune cookies
    Orange slices

Day Two
  Spinach and feta cheese omelette
  Toast
  Tuscan tuna salad (recipe follows)
  Focaccia
  1 biscotti
  Grilled salmon fillet
  Steamed asparagus spears
  Oven-roasted vegetables (recipe follows)
  Fresh fruit salad

Day Three
  1 cup whole-grain cereal with milk
  1 bowl Manhattan clam chowder or Maryland crab soup
  Large mixed green salad with olive oil and balsamic vinegar (or Essential Balance Vinaigrette, Chapter 4)
  Sourdough roll
  Broiled or grilled pork cutlet
  Braised cabbage (recipe follows)
  Baked apples (recipe follows)

Stir-Fry Chicken and Vegetables with Peanuts

  ½ cup chicken broth or water
  1 tablespoon soy sauce
  1 tablespoon oriental sesame oil
  1 teaspoon cornstarch
  ¼ teaspoon ground ginger
  2 tablespoons canola oil
  6 ounces boneless, skinless chicken breast, cut in strips

> 3 cups raw vegetables (any combination of
> carrots, Chinese cabbage, broccoli florets,
> green or red peppers, snow peas, bean
> sprouts, or other fresh vegetables) cut in
> equal-size pieces
> 2 tablespoons roasted peanuts, chopped
> 1 hardboiled egg, chopped

Combine chicken broth, soy sauce, sesame oil, cornstarch, and ginger in small bowl and set aside. Heat 1 tablespoon canola oil in wok or large skillet until hot. Add chicken and cook over high heat, stirring often, for 3 minutes or until chicken is cooked through. Remove chicken with slotted spoon and set aside. Add remaining 1 tablespoon canola oil and heat. Add hard vegetables (carrots, onion, Chinese cabbage, etc.) and cook over high heat, stirring often, for 4 to 5 minutes or until vegetables are almost done. Add soft vegetables (snow peas, peppers, bean sprouts), and cook an additional 1–2 minutes. Add chicken and broth mixture, heat briefly to thicken sauce. Serve over rice, garnished with chopped peanuts and egg. Makes two servings.

Tuscan Tuna Salad

> 4 ounces cooked tuna, fresh or canned
> ¼ cup celery, chopped
> 4–6 seedless grapes, quartered
> 1 green onion, chopped

1 tablespoon olive oil
2 teaspoons balsamic vinegar
3 large lettuce leaves, such as romaine or
endive
3–4 cherry tomatoes, halved

Break tuna into chunks but do not mash. Add celery, grapes, green onion, olive oil, and vinegar and toss lightly to mix. Arrange tuna mixture on lettuce leaves and garnish with cherry tomatoes. Makes one serving.

Oven-Roasted Vegetables

1 large sweet potato
4 small red potatoes
2 large carrots
1 tablespoon canola oil
salt to taste
caraway seeds or rosemary (optional)

Scrub but do not peel potatoes and carrots. Cut into uniform cubes, approximately 1 inch square, and place in large mixing bowl. Add canola oil and toss to coat vegetables evenly. Add salt and caraway seeds, if desired. Spread vegetables on a large baking sheet and roast in a preheated oven at 325° for 45 to 50 minutes, stirring once. (Experiment with other root vegetables, including turnips, beets, fennel, and onions.) Makes two servings.

Braised Cabbage

> ½ head green cabbage
> 1 tablespoon butter
> salt to taste

Remove the outer leaves and core of the cabbage. Cut into 1-inch strips. In a large oven-proof skillet, melt the butter (or Better Butter, Chapter 6). Add cabbage and sauté briefly until wilted and coated evenly with butter. Add salt to taste. Place skillet, uncovered, in a 325° oven and roast for 50 to 60 minutes, until cabbage is soft and lightly browned. Makes two servings.

Baked Apples

> 2 large baking apples
> 2 tablespoon raisins
> 1 tablespoon lemon juice
> 2 teaspoons sugar
> ½ teaspoon cinnamon
> ½ teaspoon grated lemon zest
> graham cracker crumbs

Wash but do not peel apples. Core and slice apples and arrange in pie pan or shallow baking dish with raisins. Sprinkle lemon juice, sugar, cinnamon, and lemon zest over fruit and bake at 350° for 40 minutes or until apples are soft. Serve warm with graham cracker crumbs sprinkled on top. Makes two servings.

Nuts and Nut Butters

Nuts provide a good source of protein and fiber in addition to essential fatty acids. A small handful of almonds makes a satisfying between-meal snack. A few roasted cashews add flavor and crunch to vegetables. Try sprinkling a few walnuts or pecans on your morning cereal for a nutritious breakfast that will take you clear through to lunch without a midmorning crash.

Nut butters are another way to enjoy the goodness of nuts, but commercial brands usually contain a lot of sugar, salt, and hydrogenated vegetable oils. Natural peanut or cashew butter is a better choice and makes a great snack spread on whole-grain toast or a few crackers.

Sources for Additional Recipes and Menu Plans

Gittleman, Ann Louise, and Dina Nunziato. *Eat Fat, Lose Weight* (Los Angeles: Keats Publishing, 1999).

Simopoulus, Artemis, M.D., and Jo Robinson. *The Omega Diet* (New York: HarperCollins, 1999).

ESSENTIAL FATS FOR NATURAL BEAUTY

In addition to being a natural weight loss aid, evening primrose oil is known for other, largely cosmetic benefits. Acne, dry skin, brittle nails, and dandruff are all classic signs of nutritional deficiency—specifically, a lack of essential fatty acids. Many women use evening primrose oil as a sort of internal beauty serum, finding that it gives them clear, fresh complexion and strong, healthy hair and nails. You might say that good health is the ultimate cosmetic.

HEALING THE SKIN

Evening primrose oil is beneficial for all types of skin disorders, including eczema (see also Chapter 5), psoriasis, and acne. As teenagers, many of us believed that oily foods made the skin more prone to acne. While adolescent acne often is aggravated by excess sebum or oil production, this is the result of changing hormone levels of adolescence, not the ingestion of dietary fats. In fact, acne often signals a deficiency of essential fatty acids.

Evening primrose oil supplements frequently can clear up long-standing complexion problems in a matter of weeks. By correcting underlying deficiencies of essential fatty acids, evening primrose oil stimulates beneficial prostaglandins that reduce swelling and inflammation. In adults, acne often is accompanied by dry skin, which can be irritated by drying acne products designed for teenage skin. The essential fatty acids in evening primrose oil helps to maintain moisture, giving the skin its supple, smooth texture.

Recommended dosage: Physicians often prescribe evening primrose oil (one to four 500-mg capsules a day) along with other nutrients to reduce acne. B vitamins, especially B_3, B_5, and B_6, support the metabolism of essential fatty acids. B_3, or niacin, improves blood flow to the skin, and people with acne often are deficient in B$_6$. Zinc helps to heal the skin tissue and prevent scarring.

RELIEF FOR DRY EYES

Decreased tear production can be a problem for contact lens wearers, allergy sufferers, and older people. Women frequently find that tear secretion diminishes after menopause. More serious is Sjögren's syndrome, an autoimmune disorder that commonly affects those with rheumatoid arthritis, causing tear and saliva production to dry up. Inadequate tear production causes the eyes to become red, irritated, and inflamed. Low saliva production can cause dental problems and contribute to poor digestion.

   Recommended dosage: Evening primrose oil (one to four 500-mg capsules a day) increases both tear and saliva production and can alleviate symptoms of Sjögren's syndrome. It also can make contact lenses more comfortable. Other helpful nutrients include vitamins A, B$_2$, B$_6$, and C.

STRONG FINGERNAILS

Changes in the fingernails can indicate nutrient deficiencies or problems in organ function, or can correspond to certain diseases. For example, thick nails can signal problems with blood circulation or thyroid disease; vertical ridges may indicate iron deficiency or kidney disorder; and bumps on the surface of the nail can result from rheumatoid arthritis. Weak, brittle fingernails are a classic indication of fatty acid deficiency. People taking evening primrose oil for other reasons have noted that the health and resilience of their fingernails improved dramatically. Other nutrients that promote healthy nails include vitamin A, vitamin D, calcium, and silica.

Recommended dosage: 1–4 500-mg capsules

HEALTHY HAIR AND SCALP

Although the hair is made up of dead tissue, hair cells are a type of skin cell, and hair loss is frequently associated with essential fatty acid deficiency. Many users of evening primrose oil report that the supplements are very effective in relieving itchy scalp and dandruff. Also recommended are vitamins B$_6$, B$_{12}$, selenium, and zinc.

Recommended dosage: 1–4 500-mg capsules

RESOURCES

Herbs and Nutritional Supplements
  L & H
  32–33 47th Avenue
  Long Island City, NY 11101
  (800) 221-1152
  (718) 361-1437
  www.bvital.com

Swanson's Health Products
P.O. Box 2803
Fargo, ND 58101
(800) 437-4148
(800) 726-7691 (fax)
www.swansonvitamins.com

VNF Nutrition
240 Route 25A
East Setauket, NY 11733
(800) 681-7099
(516) 689-7638 fax
www.vnfnutrition.com

Vitamin Shoppe
4700 Westside Avenue
North Bergen, NJ 07047
(800) 223-1216
(800) 852-7153
www.vitaminshoppe.com

Vitamin Research Products, Inc.
3579 Highway 50 East
Carson City, NV 89701
(702) 884-1300
(800) 877-2447
www.vrp.com

9

Using Evening Primrose Oil

BY now you may be so impressed with the many health-enhancing abilities of evening primrose oil that you are eager to start enjoying the benefits yourself. Before you head off to the pharmacy or health food store to purchase some supplements, you may wish to consider a few factors.

As evening primrose oil has become more popular, dozens of brands have appeared on the market, but not all are of equal quality. As you might expect, bargain-basement brands are often of inferior quality, but price is not always a reliable guide. The retail price for evening primrose oil supplements ranges from $15 to $35 for a one-month supply of 180 500-mg capsules, with reliable, high-quality brands available at both ends of the price continuum.

Efamol, Ltd., was one of the first and remains one of the largest primrose oil manufacturers in the world. It is also among the more expensive brands (although it is available for significant savings through some mail order companies). When you buy Efamol, you are assured of getting the same pharmaceutical-grade product used in most of the published research on evening primrose oil. The Efamol company, based in the United Kingdom, controls the entire process, from the breeding of the plants, to growing and harvesting techniques, all the way to the encapsulation of the product. The company owns the rights to five specific varieties of evening primrose that have been specially bred for consistent yields and potency. Efamol has also pledged to invest 35 percent of its revenue "in research to ensure the safety of their EPO products, to prove their efficacy, and to understand the mechanism of their actions."

Of course, other quality brands of evening primrose oil are available. When selecting a supplement, keep in mind several factors. First, the method used to extract the oil from the seed is of critical importance. The use of heat or chemical solvents can damage or alter the molecular structure of the fatty acids in the oil and destroy the natural antioxidants (preservatives) that keep the oil from oxidizing. Look for supplements that specify that the oils used have been cold-pressed or expeller-pressed, without chemical solvents.

It's also important that no artificial colors or preservatives have been used in the manufacture of the capsules. These additives can interfere with the absorption of the oil and block its effectiveness. In early research on evening primrose oil, scientists conducting a clinical trial on the treatment of eczema reported that no benefit was observed by those using the oil. Later it was discovered that the researchers had used a supplement that contained artificial ingredients which blocked the conversion of fatty acids in the body. Most evening primrose oil supplements contain a small amount of vitamin E as a natural antioxidant and preservative.

All fats, particularly polyunsaturated oils, are subject to spoilage if they are not handled properly. The free radicals in rancid or oxidized oils can cause significant damage in the body and should be avoided. Evening primrose oil supplements that have been properly processed should have a clean, nutty aroma and a deep golden color. You can check the freshness of the capsules by cutting them open and smelling and tasting the oil.

Evening primrose oil supplements are readily available at natural food stores, health food stores, and, increasingly, in mainstream pharmacies and grocery stores. National chains that carry evening primrose oil include Whole Foods Markets, CVS, Rite Aid, and General Nutrition Centers (GNC). In addition, you can purchase evening primrose oil through mail order companies and on the Internet.

DOSAGES

For general health maintenance and nutritional support, the most commonly recommended dosage is one to three 500-mg capsules evening primrose oil per day. Children under five can safely be given one capsule per day; two per day for children ages five to twelve. When using evening primrose oil for infants (as in the treatment of eczema), many parents find it easier to open the capsules and mix the oil with the baby's formula or food.

When dealing with serious or chronic health problems, higher amounts usually are needed. The preceding chapters include dosage recommendations based on the amounts found to be effective for those conditions in clinical trials. In general, greater therapeutic effects were seen when patients used higher dosages (eight to twelve capsules per day), but individual results can vary. It's perfectly appropriate to experiment to find the dosage that works best for you. If the recommended amount doesn't seem to help, you may wish to try increasing the dosage before giving up entirely.

As you may recall, the most potent natural source of GLA is human breast milk. For purposes of comparison, it's worth pointing out that a six-month old baby who is fully breast fed consumes up to 500 milligrams GLA each day. (The equivalent for a 150-pound adult would be 5 grams a day, or the amount found in 120 capsules of evening primrose oil!) In clinical trials, volunteers consumed up to 20 capsules a day for many months without adverse effects.

Keep in mind that, although its effects on health can be quite dramatic, evening primrose oil is not a drug and doesn't force the body to amplify or suppress any biochemical process. It simply offers a rich source of GLA, the nutritional "missing link" that our bodies need in order to optimize cellular function. Any amount of GLA in excess of what the body can use is simply metabolized and excreted. For this reason, it would be virtually impossible to overdose on evening primrose oil (although extremely high amounts would most likely cause unpleasant side effects, such as nausea or diarrhea).

You also may find that you can get good results at lower than the recommended dosages, which has benefits in terms of cost savings and convenience. Your own genetics, health history, and other dietary and nutritional factors will have a significant impact on your response. Those with an inherited inability to convert linoleic acid to GLA, as is common in those with allergies and some autoimmune disorders, probably will require more supplemental GLA in order to compensate for this metabolic problem. Other factors can interfere with this conversion, including alcohol abuse, diabetes, high cholesterol, stress, and nutrient deficiencies. Certain health conditions, such as cancer, diabetes, and viral infections, appear to increase the body's requirements for GLA. Finally, the other fats in your diet will affect your requirement and usage of GLA and other essential fatty acids. If your diet is high in trans fatty acids and saturated fats, your need for essential fatty acids will be higher than if you consume a greater percentage of your fat calories as healthy monounsaturated and polyunsaturated oils.

It can take awhile for the full effect of evening

primrose oil to become apparent. Weeks or even months of supplementation may be required to reverse long-standing deficiencies and imbalances in fatty acid metabolism. For easy reference, the accompanying chart summarizes recommended amounts of evening primrose oil for various health concerns. You will usually find evening primrose oil packaged in 500-mg capsules. See previous individual chapters for more detailed protocol information.

Recommended Dosages of Evening Primrose Oil

Condition	Daily Recommended Amount	Other Helpful Nutrients
Nutritional support and health maintenance	500–1,500 mg	B_3, B_6, C, magnesium, zinc
Alcoholism	2,000–4,000 mg	B_1, B_5, B_{12}, glutathione, C
Allergies (sinus)	2,000–4,000 mg	A, B_5, B_6, C, quercetin, zinc
Arthritis	4,000–6,000 mg	B_5, E, calcium, selenium, zinc
Asthma	2,000–6,000 mg	A, B_5, B_6, B_{12}, C, magnesium, quercetin
Diabetes	4,000–6,000 mg	B_{12}, chromium, coenzyme Q-10, L-carnitine, zinc
Eczema	4,000–6,000 mg	B_3, B_6, B_{12}, E, zinc
Food allergies	2,000–4,000 mg	B_5, B_{12}, C, glutamine, zinc, digestive enzymes

Condition	Daily Recommended Amount	Other Helpful Nutrients
Hair, skin, nails	500–2,000 mg	A, B_2, B_{12}, folic acid, biotin, calcium, silica
Heart health	2,000–4,000 mg	B_6, B_{12}, folic acid, E, coenzyme Q-10, magnesium
Multiple sclerosis	3,000–6,000 mg	B_6, B_{12}, choline, inositol, coenzyme Q-10, selenium, zinc
Premenstrual syndrome	2,000–4,000 mg	B_3, B_6, C, magnesium, zinc, calcium
Schizophrenia	4,000–6,000 mg	B_3, B_6, C, magnesium, zinc
Weight loss	2,000–4,000 mg	C, chromium, L-carnitine

Animal lovers may be interested to learn that evening primrose oil also has been used with great success to relieve itchy skin, eczema, dermatitis, and arthritis pain in dogs. Simply open one or two capsules and mix in with the dog's food once per day.

SIDE EFFECTS

Decades of research and widespread use have shown evening primrose oil to be remarkably nontoxic and well tolerated. Adverse reactions to the oil are rare and usually minor. For example, some people have reported headaches or nausea after taking evening primrose oil capsules; nausea can be avoided almost always by taking the supplements with food, not on an empty stomach. There have been occasional reports of softer stools as a result of evening primrose oil, but for many this translates into a positive side effect, namely, relief from constipation. A few users have noticed that the oil seems to make their skin oily or more prone to breakouts. (More often, however, people report that problem complexions clear up with the use of evening primrose oil.) Many of these reactions seem to be a response to the sudden introduction of unaccustomed amounts of essential fatty acids and go away with continued use. Others usually can be controlled by reducing the dosage or in building up gradually to a higher dosage.

A few situations dictate caution in the use of evening primrose oil. Large doses (twelve or more 500-mg capsules a day) have been shown to lower the seizure threshold for those suffering from temporal lobe epilepsy. Although this effect has not been seen at lower doses or with other forms of epilepsy, people with epilepsy should use evening primrose oil with caution.

Evening primrose oil may amplify the effects of several pharmaceutical drugs. Because of its beneficial effect on blood pressure, cholesterol, and blood coagulation, the use of evening primrose oil may lower the amount of drugs required to control these conditions. If you are taking anticoagulants, blood pressure drugs, or cholesterol-lowering medications, please consult a physician before adding evening primrose oil to your regimen, so that he or she can monitor your status and adjust dosages accordingly.

Likewise, the anti-inflammatory and immune-regulating effects of evening primrose oil can reduce the need for pain relievers, nonsteroidal anti-inflammatories, and other anti-inflammatory drugs in the management of arthritis, eczema, and autoimmune and inflammatory conditions. Consult a doctor before reducing or discontinuing any prescribed medications. With steroid medications in particular, it is important to taper off the drugs to avoid possible withdrawal symptoms.

PULLING IT ALL TOGETHER

In addition to evening primrose oil, there are many other ways to enjoy the health-promoting advantages of healthful fats and essential fatty acids. You can maximize the many benefits of evening primrose oil by minimizing your intake of unhealthful fats, especially trans fats, and emphasizing healthful fats in your diet.

The typical American gets 35 to 40 percent of his or her calories from fats. Here's how it breaks down:

Typical American Diet

Saturated fat (from meat and dairy products)	15%
Polyunsaturated oils	10%
Trans fatty acids (hydrogenated oils)	10%
Monounsaturated oils	3%
Total	38% of daily calorie intake

Studies have shown that we can improve our health and lower our risk of cancer and heart disease simply by making some subtle adjustments to this picture. Contrary to widely held beliefs, we don't need to reduce the total amount of fat in our diets drastically. We can enjoy these health benefits just by changing the kind of fats we eat.

Diet for Optimal Health and Longevity

Monosaturated fat (olive and canola oil)	20%
Saturated fat (from meat and dairy products)	7%
Polyunsaturated fats (including EFAs)	5%
Trans fatty acids	3% or less
Total	35% of daily calorie intake

What does this mean in terms of everyday living? You can accomplish this transformation with a few simple and delicious changes in your eating habits.

1. **Choose leaner cuts of meat.** Enjoy a lean veal or pork chop instead of fattier cuts of meat. Select extra-lean ground beef or substitute ground turkey. Opt for the breast meat in turkey and chicken rather than the fattier thigh and leg. If you do enjoy fattier types of meat, such as ground beef, ribs, or bacon, exercise portion control.

2. **Enjoy more cold-water fish,** such as salmon, herring, tuna, and cod. These healthy and delicious alternatives to meat have become so popular (especially salmon) that they are on almost every restaurant menu and available at good prices in most grocery stores.

3. **Replace full-fat dairy products with low-fat versions.** (Note: You don't need to go completely fat free. Low-fat dairy products [1 to 2 percent] cut down on saturated fat but still have a rich, satisfying taste.)

4. **Help yourself to nuts,** in moderation. With the calories you save by cutting down on saturated fats and trans fatty acids, you can enjoy more of these heart-healthy sources of monounsaturated fat without exceeding your daily fat intake.

5. **Use Better Butter** instead of butter (recipe in Chapter 6) on bread, potatoes, vegetables, and in recipes calling for shortening. Or adopt the Mediterranean custom of dipping chunks of fresh bread in extra-virgin olive oil.

6. **Use olive or canola oil** as your principal cooking oil, instead of corn or vegetable oil. (See "Tips for Buying, Storing, and Using Oils," below.) You can substitute liquid oil or a combination of oil and butter in most recipes calling for vegetable shortening.

7. **Avoid processed foods** containing hydrogenated fats, including most cookies, crackers, margarine, mayonnaise, salad dressings, chips, soup mixes, cake mixes, and so on.

Look for brands that use nonhydrogenated vegetable oils instead. Thanks to increasing awareness of the dangers of trans fats, products made without hydrogenated oil are becoming easier to find.

8. **Opt for oil-based salad dressings,** made with olive or canola oils, rather than creamy mayonnaise-based dressings. (See also the recipe for Essential Balance™ Vinaigrette in Chapter 4.) Commercial mayonnaise often is made with hydrogenated oils. The thinner consistency of vinaigrette-type dressings also helps them go further, reducing the total calorie intake.

9. **Use ripe avocado,** rich in monounsaturated fats, to add flavor and creaminess to dips and salad dressings.

10. **Round off your healthy eating plan with essential fatty acid supplements,** including evening primrose oil and fish or flaxseed oil, if you wish. Fish and flax provide essential fatty acids from the omega-3 family, which complement the beneficial actions of evening primrose oil. (See Chapter 6 for more on omega-3 fats.)

Note: Keep in mind that evening primrose oil supplements (as well as fish oil and other fatty acid supplements) count toward your total fat intake for the day. At lower dosages (two to three grams per day) the impact is minimal, contributing only a small percentage of your total fat calories. If you are using higher amounts of evening primrose oil or other fatty acid supplements for therapeutic purposes, be sure to calculate the total amount of fat provided by supplements and adjust your dietary intake accordingly.

Let's translate these principles into real terms, using a 2,000-calorie diet as an example. This is roughly the number of calories that a 150-pound person with a moderate activity level needs to maintain the weight, neither gaining nor losing.

Typical American Diet (2,000 Calories)
   Eggs and bacon, toast and butter
   Coffee with half and half
   Tuna salad sandwich
   Potato chips
   4 chocolate sandwich cookies
   Hamburger and bun
   Salad with blue cheese dressing
   Yellow cake with chocolate frosting

> Total fat equals 38 percent, or around 86 grams, including 36 grams of saturated, 28 grams of trans fats, 20 grams of monounsaturated fat, and only trace amounts of essential fatty acids.

Healthier and Just as Much Fun (2,000 Calories)
   Bagel with cream cheese
   Coffee with milk
   Grilled chicken sandwich

Pasta salad with pesto and pine nuts
Homemade brownie
Fresh roasted peanuts
Grilled salmon
Baked potato with butter
Salad with olive oil and balsamic vinegar
Angel food cake

> Total fat equals 35 percent, or around 78 grams, including 21 grams of saturated fat, 0 grams of trans fats, 35 grams of monounsaturated fats, and 13 grams essential fatty acids. The addition of four capsules of evening primrose oil brings the total essential fatty acid consumption to 15 grams, or 7 percent of the total daily intake.

As you can see, it is possible to reduce the amount of unhealthful fats in your diet without giving up anything in flavor, variety, or richness. Best of all, by reducing your consumption of saturated fat and dangerous trans fatty acids, and by increasing the amount of healthful fats in your diet, you can lower your risk of cancer and heart disease, reduce allergies and inflammation, boost your immune system, and even slow down the aging process.

Tips for Buying, Storing, and Using Oils

1. *Buy oils that are cold-pressed or expeller-processed, without chemical solvents. These oils*

retain more of the natural antioxidants that keep them fresh.

2. Choose unrefined oils that have not been heated, bleached, or had artificial preservatives added.

3. Look for oils packaged in dark glass or opaque containers that protect the contents from UV damage.

4. Store oils in a cool, dark place. Polyunsaturated oils like corn, sunflower, and grapeseed are best kept in the refrigerator. (Evening primrose oil supplements do not need to be refrigerated. The gelatin capsules protect the oil from contact with the air.)

5. Buy oil in quantities that you can use within a few weeks of opening.

6. Discard any oil that has a sour or bitter aroma or taste. The free radicals in rancid oils can cause cellular damage and should be avoided.

7. When cooking with oil, try to keep the heating time as brief as possible to protect the oil from forming harmful compounds. Sauté foods lightly instead of frying.

8. If you wish to fry foods, use peanut oil, which is the most stable oil for high temperature cooking.

9. Never reuse oil that has been heated to high temperatures.

RESOURCES

Additional Reading

Gittleman, Ann Louise, with Dina R. Nunziato.

Eat Fat, Lose Weight (Los Angeles: Keats Publishing, 1999).

Jenkins, Nancy. *The Mediterranean Diet Cookbook.* (New York: Bantam Books, 1994).

Simopoulus, Artemis, M. D., and Jo Robinson *The Omega Plan.* (New York: HarperCollins, 1998).

Mail Order and Internet Sources for Supplements

L&H
32-33 47th Avenue
Long Island City, NY 11101
(800) 221-1152
(718) 361-1437
www.bvital.com

Nature's Nutrition Store
1201 Division St
Kingston, ON K7K 6X4
(800) 238-0478
(613) 544-8535
(613) 253-6887 fax
naturesnutrition.com

Seacoast Vitamins
600 Palm Avenue, #106
Imperial Beach, CA 91932
(877) 229-1779 (toll free)
(800) 555-6792
(619) 429-1770 fax
www.seacoastvitamins.com

VNF Nutrition
240 Route 25A
East Setauket, NY 11733
(800) 681-7099
(516) 689-7638 fax
www.vnfnutrition.com

Vitamin Shoppe
4700 Westside Avenue
North Bergen, NJ 07047
(800) 223-1216
(800) 852-7153
www.vitaminshoppe.com

Vitamin Research Products, Inc.
3579 Highway 50 East
Carson City, NV 89701
(800) 877-2447
(702) 884-1300
www.vrp.com

*Manufacturers and Distributors of Evening
Primrose Oil*
American Health
4320 Veteran's Memorial Highway
Holbrook, NY 11741
(800) 445-7137
(516) 244-1777

Efamol Canada
35 Webster Street, Suite 103
Kentville, NS B4N1H4

(902) 678-2727
www.efamol.com

Health from the Sun
P.O. Box 179
Newport, NH 03773
(800) 447-2229

Nature's Plus
10 Daniel Street
Farmingdale, NY 11735
(800) 937-0500
www.naturesplus.com

Nature's Way
10 Mountain Spring Parkway
Springville, UT 84663
(800) 9-NATURE
www.naturesway.com

Now Foods
395 South Glenellyn
Bloomingdale, IL 60108
(800) 999-8069
www.nowfoods.com

Spectrum Naturals
133 Copeland Street
Petaluma, GA 94952
(808) 778-8900

Sources for High-Quality Oils

Arrowhead Mills (a division of Hain Foods)
P.O. Box 2059
Hereford, TX 79045
(800) 749-0730

Barlean's Organic Oils
4936 Lake Terrell Road
Ferndale, WA 98248
(800) 445-3529
www.barleans.com

Food and Vine Inc.
301 Poplar Avenue, Suite 6
Mill Valley, CA 94941
(888) 388-7117
www.grapeseedoil.com

Omega Nutrition
6515 Aldrich Road
Bellingham, WA 98226
(800) 661-3529
(360) 384-0700
www.omegaflo.com

Spectrum Naturals
133 Copeland Street
Petaluma, GA 94952
(808) 778-8900

References

Books

Balch, James, M.D. and Phyllis Balch. *Prescription for Nutritional Healing*. Garden City Park, NY: Avery Publishing Group, 1997.

Barilla, Jean, M.S., ed. *The Good Fats & Oils*. New Canaan, CT: Keats Publishing, 1996.

Cass, Hyla, M.D. *St. John's Wort: Nature's Blues Buster*. Garden City Park, NY: Avery Publishing Group, 1998.

Conkling, Winifred. *Secrets of 5-HTP*. New York: St. Martin's Press, 1998.

Gittleman, Ann Louise, M.S., C.N.S. *Eat Fat, Lose Weight*. Los Angeles: Keats Publishing, 1999.

Graham, Judy, *Evening Primrose Oil: Its Remarkable Properties and Its Use in the Treatment of a Wide Range of Conditions*. Rochester, VT: Healing Arts Press, 1989.

Haas, Elson M., M.D. *Staying Healthy with Nutrition*. Berkeley, CA: Celestial Arts Publishing, 1992.

Hoffman, Ronald L. *Intelligent Medicine*. New York: Fireside, 1997.

Lark, Susan M., M.D. *Premenstrual Syndrome Self-Help Book*. Berkeley, CA: Celestial, 1984.

Lark, Susan M., M.D. *Women's Health Companion: Self-Help Nutrition Guide and Cookbook*. Berkeley, CA: Celestial Arts Publishing, 1995.

Rosenbaum, Michael, M.D., and Dominick Bosco. *Super Supplements*. New York: Signet, 1989.

Simopoulos, Artemis, M.D. *The Omega Plan*. New York: HarperCollins, 1989.

Walji, Hasnain, Ph.D. *Evening Primrose Oil*. London: Thorsons, 1996.

Articles

Abraham, G. E. "Nutritional Factors in the Etiology of the Premenstrual Tension Syndromes." *Journal of Reproductive Medicine* 28, no. 7 (July 1983): 446–464

Abraham, R. D. "Effects of Safflower Oil and Evening Primrose Oil, in Men with a Low Dihomo-gamma-linolenic Level." *Atherosclerosis* 81, no. 3 (April 1990): 199–208

Allred, J. D. "An Overemphasis on Eating Low-Fat Foods May Be Contributing to the Alarming Increase in Overweight." *Journal of the American Dietetic Association* 95, no. 4 (1995): 417–18.

Asherio, A., et al. "Health Effects of Trans Fatty Acids." *American Journal of Clinical Nutrition* 66, 4 Suppl, (October 1997): 1006S–1010S.

Belch, J. J., et al. "Effects of Altering Dietary Essential Fatty Acids on Requirements for Non-Steroidal Anti-

Inflammatory Drugs in Patients with Rheumatoid Arthritis." *Annals of Rheum Dis* 47, no. 2 (February 1988): 96–104.

Belch, J. J., et al. "Evening Primrose Oil in the Treatment of Raynaud's Phenomenon." *Thromb Haemot* 54, no.2 (August 1985): 490–494.

Berger, P. A. "Biochemistry and the Schizophrenia." *Journal of Nervous and Mental Dis* 169, no. 2 (February 1981): 90–99.

Berth-Jones, J., and R. A. Graham-Brown. "Placebo-Controlled Trial of Essential Fatty Acid Supplementation in Atopic Dermatitis." *Lancet* 341, no. 8860 (June 1993): 1557–1560.

Berth-Jones, J., et al. "Evening Primrose Oil and Atopic Eczema." *Lancet* 345 (January 1995): 520.

Biagi, P. L. "A Long-Term Study on the Use of Evening Primrose Oil in Atopic Children." *Drugs Exp Clin Res* 14, no. 4 (1988): 285–290.

Booyens, J., et al. "Some Effects of the Essential Fatty Acids on the Proliferation of Human Osteogenic Sarcoma Cells in Culture." *Prostaglandins Leukot Med* 15, no. 1 (July 1984): 15–33.

Bordoni, A., et al. "Evening Primrose Oil in the Treatment of Children with Atopic Eczema." *Drugs Exp Clin Res* 14, no. 4 (1988): 291–297.

Brzeski, M., et al. "Evening Primrose Oil in Patients with Rheumatoid Arthritis and Side Effects of Non-Steroidal Anti-Inflammatory Drugs." *Br J Rheumatol* 30, no. 5 (October 1991): 370–372.

Bunce, O. R. "Eicosanoid Synthesis and Ornithine Decarboxylase Activity in Mammary Tumors of Rats Fed Varying Levels and Types of n-3 and/or n-6 Fatty

Acids." *Prostaglandins Leukot Essent Fatty Acids* 41, no. 2 (October 1999): 105–113.

Caggiula, A. W. "Effects of Dietary Fat and Fatty Acids on Coronary Artery Disease Risk." *American Journal of Clinical Nutrition* 65, 5 Suppl. (May 1997): 1597S–1610S.

Callender, K., et al. "A Double-Blind Trial of Evening Primrose Oil in the Premenstrual Syndrome." *Human Psychopharm* 3 (1988): 57–61.

Cameron, N. E. "Metabolic and Vascular Factors in the Pathogenesis of Diabetic Neuropathy." *Diabetes* 46, Suppl. 2 (September 1997): S31–37.

Charalambous, B. M. "Erythrocyte Sodium Pump Activity in Human Obesity." *Clin Chim Acta* 141, no. 2–3 (August 1984): 179–187.

Claassen, N., et al. "The Effect of Different n-6/n-3 Fatty Acid Ratios on Calcium Balance and Bone In rats." *Prostaglandins Leukot Essent Fatty Acids* 53, no. 1 (July 1995): 13–19.

Corbett, R. "The Effects of Chronic Administration of Ethanol on Synaptosomal Fatty Acid Composition." *Alcohol Alcohol* 27, no. 1 (January 1992): 11–14.

Crawford, M. A., et al. "Comparative Studies on the Metabolic Equivalence of Linoleic and Arachidonic Acids." *Nutr Metab* 21, Suppl. 1 (1977): 189–190.

De Luise M. "Reduced Activity of the Red-Cell Sodium-Potassium Pump in Human Obesity." *New England Journal of Medicine* 303, no. 18 (October 1980): 1017–1122.

Dines, K. C. "Effectiveness of Natural Oils as Sources of GLA to Correct Peripheral Nerve Conduction."

Prostaglandins Leukot Essent Fatty Acids 55, no. 3 (September 1996): 159–165.

Duffy, O. "Attenuation of the Effects of Ethanol in the Brain Lipid Content of the Developing Rate by an Oil Enriched in Gamma-Linoleic Acid. *Drug Alcohol Depend* 31, no. 1 (October 1992): 85–89.

Duffy, O. "Effects of an Oil Enriched in GLA on Locomotor Activity and Behaviour in the Morris Maze." *Drug Alcohol Depend* 30, no. 1 (April 1992): 65–70.

Ebden, P., et al. "A Study of Evening Primrose Seed Oil in Atopic Asthma." *Prostaglandins Leukot Essent Fatty Acids* 35, no. 2 (February 1989): 69–72.

El-Ela, S. H., et al. "Effects of Dietary Primrose Oil on Mammary Tumorogenesis." *Lipids* 22, no. 12 (December 1987): 1041–1044.

Fried, L. P., et al. "Risk Factors for 5-Year Mortality in Older Adults." *Journal of the American Medical Association* 25, no. 8 (February 1998): 585–592.

Fuller, C. J. "Effects of Antioxidants and Fatty Acids on LDL Oxidation." *American Journal of Clinical Nutrition* 60, 6 Suppl. (December 1994): 1010S–1013S.

Gately, C. A., et al. "Drug Treatments for Mastalgia: 17 Years Experience in the Cardiff Mastalgia Clinic." *Journal of the Royal Society of Medicine* 85, no. 1 (January 1992): 12–15.

Golay, A., et al. "Weight Loss with a Low or High Carbohydrate Diet." *International Journal of Obesity* 20 (1996): 1062–1072.

Goodwin, P. J., M. Neelam, and N. F. Boyd. "Cyclical Mastopathy: A Critical Review of Therapy." *British Journal of Surgery* 75 (September 1988): 837–844.

Grundy, S. M. "What Is the Desirable Ratio of Fatty Acids in the Diet?" *American Journal of Clinical Nutrition* 44, 4 Suppl. (October 1997): 988S–990S.

Hansen, T. M. "Treatment of Rheumatoid Arthritis with Prostaglandin E1 Precursors Cis-Linoleic Acid and Gamma-Linoleic Acid." *Scand J Rheumatol* 12, no. 2 (1983): 85–88.

Hassam A. G. "Incorporation of Gamma-Linolenic Acid and Linoleic Acid into the Liver and Brain Lipids of Suckling Rats." *Lipids* 10 no. 7 (July 1975): 417–420.

Hassam, A. G., et al. "Potency of GLA in Curing Essential Fatty Acid Deficiency in the Rat." *Nutr Metab*, 21 Suppl 1 (1977): 190–192.

Hederos, C. A. "Epogam Evening Primrose Oil in Atopic Dermatitis and Asthma." *Archives of Diseases of Child* 75, no. 6 (December 1996): 494–497.

Holmes, M. D. "Association of Dietary Intake of Fat and Fatty Acids with Risk of Breast Cancer." *Journal of the American Medical Association*, 281, no. 10 (March 1999): 914–920.

Horrobin, D. F. "Abnormalities in Plasma Essential Fatty Acid Levels in Women with Premenstrual Syndrome and with Nonmalignant Breast Disease." *J Nutr Med* 2 (1991): 259–264.

Horrobin, D. F. "The Effects of Evening Primrose Oil, Safflower Oil and Paraffin on Plasma Fatty Acid Levels in Humans." *Prostaglandins Leukot Essent Fatty Acids* 42, no. 4 (April 1991): 245–249.

Horrobin, D. F. "Essential Fatty Acid and Prostaglandin Metabolism in Sjogren's Syndrome, Systemic Sclerosis and Rheumatoid Arthritis." *Scand J Rheumatol Suppl* 61 (1986): 242–245.

Horrobin, D. F. "Nutritional and Medical Importance of Gamma-Linolenic acid." *Prog Lipid Res* 31, no. 2 (1992): 163–194.

Horrobin, D. F. "Schizophrenia: The Role of Abnormal Essential Fatty Acid and Prostaglandin Metabolism." *Med Hypotheses* 10, no. 3 (March 1983): 329–336.

Horrobin, D. F. "The Relationship between Schizophrenia and Essential Fatty Acid on Eicosanoid Metabolism." *Prostaglandins Leukot Essent Fatty Acids* 46, no. 1 (May 1992): 71–77.

Horrobin, D. F. "The Role of Essential Fatty Acids and Prostaglandins in the Premenstrual Syndrome." *J Reprod Med* 28, no. 7 (July 1983): 465–468.

Horrobin, D. F., and P. F. Morse. "Evening Primrose Oil and Atopic Eczema." *Lancet* 345 (January 1995): 260–261.

Horrobin, D. F. et al. "Essential Fatty Acids in Plasma Phospholipids in Schizophrenics." *Biological Psychiatry* 25, no. 5 (March 1989): 562–568.

Horrobin D. F., et al. "Fatty Acid Levels in the Brains of Schizophrenics and Normal Controls." *Biol Psychiatry* 30, no. 8 (October 1991): 795–805.

Hounsom, L. "A Lipoic Acid-Gammalinolenic Acid Conjugate Is Effective Against Multiple Indices of Experimental Diabetic Neuropathy." *Diabetologia* 41, no. 7 (July 1998): 839–843.

Hu, F. B. "Dietary Fat Intake and the Risk of Coronary Heart Disease." *New England Journal of Medicine* 377, no. 21 (November 1997): 1491–1499.

Hudson, T. "Essential Fatty Acids and Women's Health—Part I." *Townsend Letter of Doctors and Patients*, 185 (December 1998): 139–141.

Hunter, D. J. "Cohort Studies of Fat Intake and the Risk of Breast Cancer." *New England Journal of Medicine* 334, no. 6 (February 1996): 356–361.

Ishikawa, T. "Effects of GLA on Plasma Lipoproteins and Apoliproteins." *Atherosclerosis* 75, no. 2–3 (February 1989): 95–104.

James, W. P. T. "Thermogenesis and Obesity." *British Medical Bulletin* 37 (1981): 43–48.

Jantti, J., et al. "Evening Primrose Oil in Rheumatoid Arthritis: Changes in Serum Lipids and Fatty Acids." *Ann Rheum Dis* 48, no. 2 (February 1989): 124–127.

Jialal, I. "Effect of Vitamin E, Vitamin C and Beta-Carotene on LDL Oxidation." *Canadian Journal of Cardiology* 11, Suppl. G (October 1995): 97G–103G.

Katan, M. B. "Trans Fatty Acids and Their Effects on Lipoproteins in Humans." *Annual Review of Nutrition* 15 (1995): 473–493.

Kronmal, R. A. "Total Serum Cholesterol Levels and Mortality Risk." *Archives of Internal Medicine*, 153, no. 9 (May 1993): 1065–1073.

Kruger, M. C., et al. "Calcium, Gamma-Linolenic Acid and Eicosapentaenoic Acid Supplementation in Senile Osteoporosis." *Agins (Milano)* 10, no. 5 (October 1998): 385–394.

Kruger, M. C. "Calcium Metabolism, Osteoporosis and Essential Fatty Acids." *Prog Lipid Res* 36, no. 2–3 (September 1997): 131–151.

Larsson, B., A. Jonason, and S. Fianu. "Evening Primrose Oil in the Treatment of Premenstrual Syndrome: A Pilot Study." *Current Ther Res* 46, no. 1 (July 1989): 58–63.

Leichsenring, M., et al. "Omega-6 Fatty Acids in Plasma Lipids of Children with Atopic Bronchial Asthma." *Pediatr Allergy Immunol* 6, no. 4 (November 1995): 209–212.

Leventhal, L. J., et al. "Treatment of Rheumatoid Arthritis with Gammalinolenic Acid." *Annals of Internal Medicine* 1, no. 9 (November 1993): 867–873.

Manku, M. S., et al. "Reduced Levels of Prostaglandin Precursors in the Blood of Atopic Patients." *Prostaglandins Leukotrienes and Medicine* 9 (1982): 615–628.

Manthorpe, R., et al. "Primary Sjogren's Syndrome Treated with Efamol/Efavit. A Double-Blind Cross-Over Investigation." *Rheumatol Int* 4, no. 4 (1984): 165–167.

Meehan, E., et al. "Influence of an n-6 Polyunsaturated Fatty-Acid Enriched Diet on the Development of Tolerance During Chronic Ethanol Administration in Rats." *Alcohol Clin Exp Res* 19, no. 6 (Dec 1995): 1441–1446.

Mercer, S. W. "Effect of High Fat Diets on Energy Balance and Thermogenesis in Brown Adipose Tissue of Lean and Genetically Obese Mice." *Journal of Nutrition* 117, no. 12 (December 1987): 2147–2153.

Morse, P. F., et al. "Meta-Analysis of Placebo-Controlled Studies of the Efficacy of Epogam in the Treatment of Atopic Eczema." *British Journal of Dermatology* 121 (1989): 75–90.

Munoz, S. E. "Differential Modulation by Dietary n-6 or n-9 Unsaturated Fatty Acids on the Development of Two Murine Mammary Gland Tumors." *Cancer Lett* 126, no. 2 (April 1998): 149–155.

Ockerman, P., et al. "Evening Primrose Oil as a Treatment of the Premenstrual Syndrome." *Rec Adv Clin Nutr* 2 (1986): 404–405.

Osler, P. "Blood Pressure and Adipose Tissue Linoleic Acid." *Res Exp Med* 175 (1979): 287–291.

Oxholm, P., et al. "Essential Fatty Acid Status in Cell Membranes and Plasma of Patients with Primary Sjogren's Syndrome." *Prostaglandins Leukot Essent Fatty Acids* 59, no. 4 (October 1998): 239–245.

Oxholm, P., et al. "Patients with Primary Sjogren's Syndrome Treated for Two Months with Evening Primrose Oil." *Scand J Rheumatol* 15, no. 2 (1986): 103–108.

Parthasarathy, S. "HDL Inhibits the Oxidative Modification of LDL." *Biochim Biophys Acta* 1044, no. 2 (May 1990): 275–283.

Preece, P. E., et al. "Evening Primrose Oil (Efamol) for Mastalgia." In Horrobin, D. F., ed. *Clinical Use of Essential Fatty Acids*. Montreal: Eden Press, 1982, 147–52.

Pritchard, G. A. "Lipids in Breast Carcinogenesis." *British Journal of Surgery* 76, no. 10 (October 1989): 1069–1073.

Puolakka, J., et al. "Biochemical and Clinical Effects of Treating the Premenstrual Syndrome with Prostaglandin Synthesis Precursors." *Journal of Reproductive Medicine* 30 (1985): 149–153.

Ramesh, G. "Effect of Evening Primrose and Fish Oils

on Two Stage Skin Carcinogenesis in Mice." *Prostaglandins Leukot Essent Fatty Acids* 59, no. 3 (September 1998): 155–161.

Ramesh, G. "Effect of Fatty Acids on Tumor Cells." *Nutrition* 8, no. 5 (September–October 1992): 343–347.

Reaven, P., et al. "Effects of Oleate-Rich and Linoleate-Rich Diets on the Susceptibility of LDL to Oxidative Modification." *J Clin Invest* 91, no. 2 (February 1993): 668–676.

Renaud, S. "Comparative Beneficial Effects on Platelet Functions and Atherosclerosis of Dietary Linoleic and Gamma-Linolenic Acids in the Rabbit." *Atherosclerosis* 45, no. 1 (October 1982): 43–51.

Renaud, S. "Cretan Mediterranean Diet for Prevention of Coronary Heart Disease." *American Journal of Clinical Nutrition* 61, 6 Suppl. (June 1995): 1360S–1367S.

Rossner, S. "Fatty Acid Composition in Serum Lipids and Adipose Tissue in Severe Obesity Before and After Six Weeks of Weight Loss. *International Journal of Obesity* 13, no. 5 (1989): 603–612.

Rouse, L. R., et al "Effects of Isoenergetic, Low-Fat Diets on Energy Metabolism in Lean and Obese Women." *American Journal of Clinical Nutrition* 60 (1994): 470–475.

Schlundt, D. "Randomized Evaluation of a Lowfat Diet for Weight Reduction." *International Journal of Obesity* 17 (1993): 623–629.

Siliprandi, N. "Significance of Evening Primrose Oil in the Problem of Nutritional Value of Poly-Unsaturated Fatty Acids." *Minerva Dietol Gastroenterol* 35, no. 1 (January–March 1989): 39–45.

Sugano, M. "Hypocholesterolemic Effect of Gamma-Linolenic Acid as Evening Primrose Oil In Rats." *Ann Nutr Metab* 30, no. 5 (1986): 289–299.

Taylor, W. C. "Cholesterol Reduction and Life Expectancy." *Annals of Internal Medicine* 106, no. 4 (April 1987): 605–614.

Tzonou, A. "Diet and Coronary Heart Disease." *Epidemiology* 4, no. 6 (November 1993): 511–516.

Vaddadi, K. S. "A Double-Blind Trial of Essential Fatty Acid Supplementation in Patients with Tardive Dyskinesia." *Psychiatry Research* 27, no. 3 (March 1989): 313–323.

Vaddadi, K. S. "Penicillin and Essential Fatty Acid Supplementation in Schizophrenia." *Prostaglandins Med* 2, no. 1 (January 1979): 77–80.

Vaddadi, K. S. "Use of GLA in the Treatment of Schizophrenia and Tardive Dyskinesia." *Prostaglandins Leukot Essent Fatty Acids* 46, no. 1 (May 1992): 67–70.

Vaddadi, K. S., and D. F. Horrobin. "Weight Loss Produced by Evening Primrose Oil Administration in Normal and Schizophrenic Individuals." *IRCS Journal of Medical Science* 7 (1979): 52.

Vaddadi, K. S., et al. "Fatty Acids. *Schizophrenia Research* 20, no. 3 (July 1996): 287–294.

Van Kammen, D. P., et al. "Polyunsaturated Fatty Acids, Prostaglandins, and Schizophrenia." *Annals of the New York Academy of Sciences* 559 (1989): 411–423.

Varma, P. K. "Protection Against Ethanol-Induced Embryonic Damage by Administering GLA and Linoleic Acids." *Prostaglandins Leukot Med* 8, no. 6 (June 1982): 641–645.

Willett, W. C. "Intake of Trans Fatty Acids and Risk of Coronary Heart Disease Among Women." *Lancet* 341, no. 8845 (March 1993): 581–585.

Wright, S. "Atopic Dermatitis and Essential Fatty Acids." *Acta Derm Venereol (Stockh)* Suppl. 114 (1985): 143–145.

Wright, S., and J. L. Burton. "Oral Evening Primrose Seed Oil Improves Atopic Eczema." *Lancet* 2 (November 1982): 1120–1122.

Wurtman, J. J. "Nutritional Intervention in Premenstrual Syndrome." In Smith, S., ed., *Modern Management of Premenstrual Syndrome.* New York: Norton Medical Books, 1983: 101–108.

Zock, P. L., and M. B. Katan. "Trans Fatty Acids, Lipoproteins, and Coronary Risk." *Can J Physiol Pharmacol* 75, no. 3 (March 1997): 211–216.

About the Author

Monica Reinagel is a freelance writer and editor, specializing in nutrition and alternative and complementary medicine. She lives in Baltimore, Maryland.